Low Cholesterol Cookbook

**1000 days** **of healthy recipes to manage blood cholesterol levels and live a healthy life, with a 30-day meal plan**

By

Diana Martinez

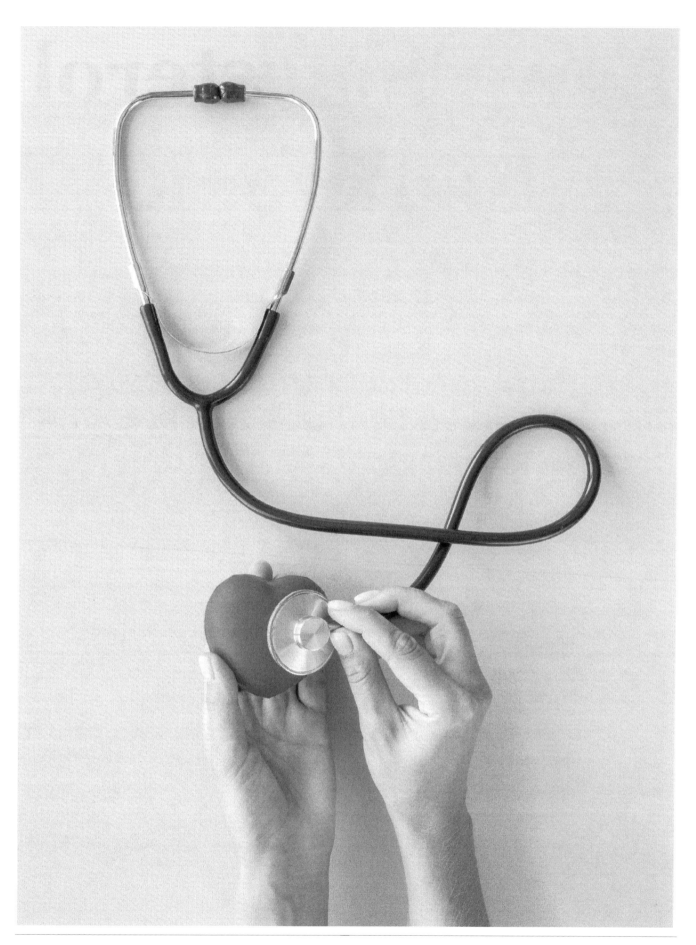

TABLE OF CONTENT

Introduction

Cholesterol and its impact on the body, particularly the heart, are complex. This book explains the many components and factors and explains what you can do to lower your cholesterol and improve your health. The foods you consume and the manner you exercise your body have a major influence on your health.

Cholesterol is a chemical distributed throughout the body in the walls of our cells. It is needed to produce key hormones. Fat is essential for transporting nutrients, maintaining a constant body temperature, protecting organs and providing quick energy. You may grow wearier, acquire more infections and diseases, and become lacking in vitamins and minerals if you do not consume enough fat. If our bodies have too much cholesterol, part of it might become stuck in the artery walls and obstruct our blood vessels. The blood may not provide the heart with enough oxygen when this occurs.

The blood cholesterol levels can be easily reduced by making a few simple changes. The best part is that foods that lower cholesterol and triglycerides are tasty and simple to prepare. Diets can be too low in fat, believe it or not.

If your blood cholesterol is high, you're more likely to have a heart attack, the leading cause of death. The good news is that you can make efforts to lower your cholesterol and make it more manageable.

Over time you may experience chest pain, which could lead to a heart attack. This condition is more common in men over 45 and women over 55. Heart attacks are also increased by unhealthy habits such as smoking, overeating and lack of physical activity.

It's critical to consume the proper fat in the right amounts. Many recipes in this book have less than 100 mg of cholesterol.

Meat, eggs, and dairy foods are high in saturated fats, which cause a significant rise in cholesterol. Some vegetable oils, palm oil, and coconut oil are rich in cholesterol oil, so keep an eye on them. Total cholesterol levels of less than 200 mg/dl are desirable, whereas cholesterol levels of 200 to 239 mg/dl are considered borderline. Because the numbers frequently vary, having a blood test regularly is the best method to keep track of one's cholesterol levels. Expert nutritionists recommend that you restrict your daily total fat consumption to less than 20% of your total daily calorie intake, total saturated fat intake to less than 7% of your daily fat intake, and daily trans-fat intake to less than 1% of your daily fat intake to maintain your blood cholesterol low. Monounsaturated fats from nuts, seeds, seafood, and vegetable oils should be included in your diet as much as possible. Other foods with little or no fat, such as whole grains, potatoes, fruits, and vegetables, may provide your body with critical vitamins and mineral requirements.

Before modifying your diet or adding exercise, consult your doctor, as with any health and nutrition recommendations. You'll have a better chance of living a healthy life if you eat a balanced diet, exercise regularly, and don't smoke.

Chapter 1: Cholesterol and Your Health

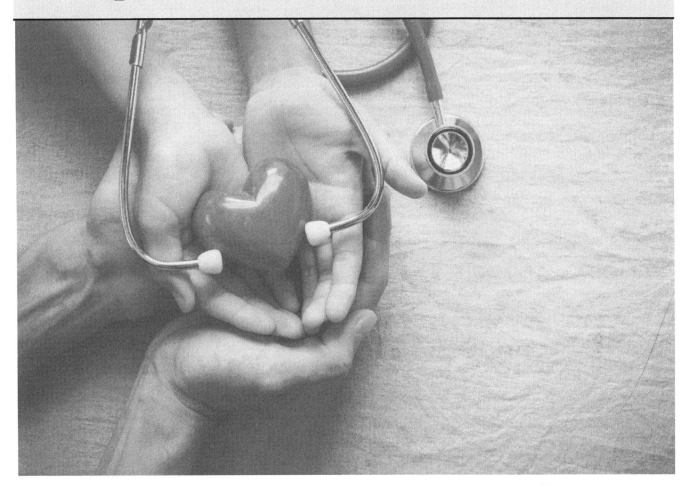

A healthy diet may greatly impact your cholesterol levels and heart health, whether your cholesterol has crept up over the years or you have an inherited problem. It will also benefit your health in other ways, including lowering blood pressure, avoiding diabetes, and helping you maintain a healthy weight. The topic of decreasing cholesterol appears to be on everyone's mind these days. It's become a regular topic of conversation, with stories about it in your local newspaper and advertisements for treatments on television. Maybe you're reading this book because your doctor said your cholesterol was "high" or "borderline." These phrases seem to be flung about all the time. Perhaps you already have heart or vascular issues that are made worse by high cholesterol. Maybe you're just attempting to eat a heart-healthy diet. Whatever the case may be, you're likely to have concerns such as:

- What is cholesterol, and how high does it have to be before it becomes an issue?
- Why is there so much debate about good and bad cholesterol?
- What dietary and lifestyle adjustments are required to decrease cholesterol?

This book answers all your queries and mentions ways to lower your cholesterol primarily from a dietary standpoint because, after all, this is a cookbook. You should always talk to your doctor or other health care provider if you have medical questions.

1.1 What Is Cholesterol?

Cholesterol is a waxy substance made up of two acetate molecules joined together. It's found in animals since the liver produces it. Cholesterol is not found in plants. The body needs cholesterol to produce hormones and steroids, as well as cell membranes. We need cholesterol to survive.

However, the amount of cholesterol in our bodies and the balance between the two types of cholesterol and other molecules such as homocysteine, triglycerides, and free radicals can anticipate whether we are at risk for atherosclerosis, heart disease, and stroke. Too much of the wrong kind of cholesterol might raise your chances of becoming sick And the way cholesterol interacts with other chemicals in the body also increases the risk of disease.

1.2 Causes and Symptoms

Both genetic and dietary factors cause cholesterol. If your parents or grandparents had high cholesterol, there's a good chance you'll have it as well. Physicians don't know whether the increased risk is due to genetics or if individuals who have unhealthy eating habits in their parents prefer to eat the same way, implying that even inherited risk might be partially due to diet. However, nutrition has a significant role in cholesterol levels. Saturated fats are the main problem in our diets. Unfortunately, many foods people like eating, such as fatty meats, fried meals, high-fat dairy products like whole milk, cream, and cheese produced from whole milk, and commercial baked goods, are rich in saturated fats.

Most of the time, high cholesterol has no symptoms. In most cases, it only results in emergencies. Damage induced by excessive cholesterol, for example, may result in a heart attack or stroke.

These instances normally don't occur until plaque builds up in your arteries due to high cholesterol levels. Plaque may restrict arteries, enabling less blood to flow through. Plaque changes your artery lining structure, which might have serious consequences.

Only a blood test can tell you whether your cholesterol is too high. A total blood cholesterol level of more than 240 mg/dl is considered high. After you turn 20, ask your doctor to perform a cholesterol test. Then, every 4 to 6 years, get your cholesterol checked again.

1.3 Good and Bad Cholesterol

When your doctor does a blood test to confirm your cholesterol levels, he looks for a few things. These are cholesterol subcomponents, and they are not the same when it comes to your health. The three most often evaluated are low-density lipoproteins (HDL), high-density lipoproteins (HDL), and triglycerides. These cholesterol components in a deciliter of blood are measured in milligrams per deciliter (mg/dl). Let's take a look at each one individually. LDL is a kind of cholesterol frequently referred to as "bad cholesterol." The portion of your total cholesterol is most responsible for clogging your arteries.

When LDL adheres to the inner surface of an artery, it promotes inflammation, which stimulates the deposit of additional cholesterol, increasing the risk of a blockage or blood clot. A primary cause of a rise in LDL is eating meals rich in saturated fats. Although the exact quantity of LDL that causes a risk is still debated, everyone knows that anything over 200 mg/dl is harmful. Even amounts above 100 mg/dl, according to some experts, may raise your risk of heart attack and stroke, depending on the source and other risk factors (such as smoking and being overweight).

HDL is often referred to as "good cholesterol." HDL assists the body in removing cholesterol deposits from the arteries. A high HDL level means you're less likely to have a heart attack. Men should have at least 40 mg/dl HDL, and women should have at least 50 mg/dl HDL. The good news is that lowering your LDL levels tends to improve your HDL levels. Adding good fat to your diet can also help you raise HDL levels. Some sources include fatty fish like tuna and salmon, olive and canola oil, and the oils found in nuts and soybeans. Some studies even claim that consuming a modest quantity of alcohol raises HDL levels.

Triglycerides are the third significant component of a typical cholesterol test. Triglycerides, like LDL, may cause a buildup of deposits in the arteries. They, like LDL, are elevated by a high-saturated-fat diet. Triglyceride levels of less than 150 mg/dl are suggested. It's worth noting that some physicians feel the ratio between HDL and LDL is even more crucial than the individual figures. As a result, whatever people do to reduce LDL and boost HDL impacts this ratio.

Chapter 2: Risk Factors of high cholesterol

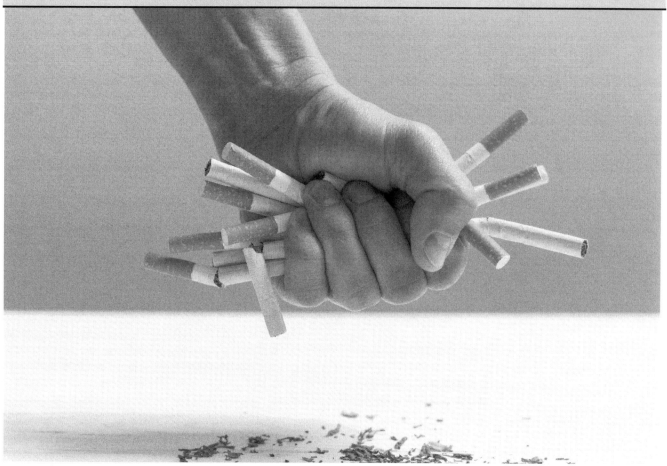

Heart disease risk factors fluctuate from person to person. Some persons may have high HDL/LDL ratios an\d blood cholesterol levels despite consuming a lot of saturated fats and cholesterol. Others have a hostile response to food and develop complications soon. To combat the condition with the right balance of diet, exercise, and prescription drugs, it's critical to first recognize your particular risk factors.

Family History

One of the most important indicators or predictors of developing heart disease is family history. The amount of cholesterol your body generates each day is regulated by your genes. You can't change your genes, but you can improve your health by treating your body well. Your liver generates between 800 and 1000 milligrams of cholesterol every day, significantly more than you can consume. Because cholesterol is a necessary component of life, your body ensures that you always have enough. You don't need to consume any cholesterol; your body produces enough to keep you healthy. Familial hypercholesterolemia is a genetic abnormality that causes the body to naturally create higher LDL cholesterol, despite diet and exercise. To help regulate cholesterol levels, people with this mutation must typically rely on prescription medicines.

Smoking

Smoking is not allowed. If you smoke, you should try to quit as soon as possible because it raises LDL cholesterol and lowers HDL cholesterol, and inflammation is also a consequence. Cigarette smoke includes about 4,000 chemicals, including at least 43 carcinogens classified as class C. It also boosts the clotting mechanism in the blood, leading to thrombosis, heart attack, or stroke.

Trans Fats Consumption

Trans fats are artificial food made by mixing hydrogen atoms with polyunsaturated fats. The body does not recognize the resulting molecule as a foreign object, and it is incorporated into everything from cell membranes to hormones. This affects your health by altering the function of certain parts of your body. Trans fats enhance the amount of LDL cholesterol and should be strictly avoided. Consume many fresh foods, such as fruits, lean meats, dairy products, whole grains, and veggies. But, learn to read labels and avoid processed and quick meals, even if the label says, "0 g trans-fat per serving," if the word hydrogenated appears in the ingredient list, the food contains trans-fat.

Sedentary Lifestyle

Even including mild to moderate exercise into your weekly routine will help lower LDL cholesterol and raise HDL levels. The American Heart Association suggests thirty minutes of moderate exercise five times each week. However, you do not have to work out for thirty minutes in a row. For the same health benefit, break it up into three ten-minute sessions. Before starting an exercise regimen, be sure you have your doctor's approval. Begin slowly. After a tough exercise, nothing destroys your determination like very painful muscles. Your objective is to be able to work out the next day.

You will have health issues if your cholesterol level is too low. Low cholesterol levels may cause depression and anxiety because serotonin levels in the brain are reduced. People with extremely low cholesterol levels (below 100 mg/dL) are more likely to have suicidal thoughts and violence.

Obesity

Maintain or improve a healthy weight and BMI. Compare your height to the weight ranges on charts provided by insurance companies. Overweight is defined as carrying more than 20% of your body weight over the highest weight for your height. Obesity is defined as a proportion of your bodyweight exceeding 30%.

Sodium

People consume much too much sodium in their diets. One issue is that salt is included in many processed meals and restaurant cuisine. This "invisible" salt is often sufficient to fulfill our daily needs. It's tough to cut salt out of your diet since it's naturally found in many foods and is utilized in large amounts in processed meals. Read labels carefully and keep track of how much sodium you ingest in a day. The entire number will surprise you!

If you truly like the taste of salt, consider sprinkling a tiny quantity on your dish just before you eat it. The salt will contact your taste receptors rapidly in this manner, making the meal taste saltier. Salt can be replaced by herbs, spices, and acidic components like lemon and vinegar. According to studies, people who eat a low-salt diet have a 20% reduced risk of heart disease and a 20% lower risk of dying from a heart attack. It will take some time and effort to switch to a low-salt diet. This may be tough at first since our taste receptors are used to salt; in fact, people begin to want salt as early as four months of life. However, after a time, you'll notice that less salt makes meals taste better, and many processed items will taste overly salty.

Poor Diet

A diet high in processed foods and low in fruits and vegetables leads to the development of heart disease. People prefer fast foods and highly processed foods to save time due to their hectic lives. Our health has suffered as we have moved away from whole foods.

Chapter 3: Structured Diet to Cure Cholesterol

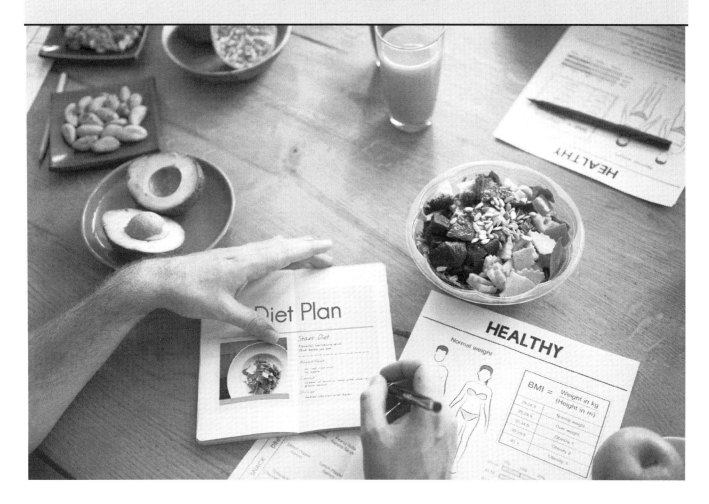

Your cholesterol and overall heart health are affected by a variety of things. Some of these, such as genetics and age, are beyond your control. Others, on the other hand, you do. Lowering cholesterol may be accomplished in three ways when it comes down to it. One is medication, which you should discuss with your doctor. Exercising is another option. Regular exercise has been demonstrated in studies to decrease cholesterol and lessen the risk of heart disease and stroke. Many cardiologists advocate at least 30 minutes of walking every day. It isn't tough, but it does need dedication.

As previously stated, the third step is to reduce the quantity of saturated fat in your diet. The good news is that the quantity of saturated fat is now mandated to be included on nutrition labels, making it quite simple to keep track of. However, saturated fat isn't the only unhealthy fat. Trans fatty acids, often known as trans fats, are created by hydrogenating liquid fat to make it solid at room temperature, as in margarine. Trans fats are now included on the nutrition labels of packaged goods, making it easy to keep track of them. If trans fats aren't stated in the nutritional information, such as in a recipe, you may determine them by subtracting total fat from saturated fat, monounsaturated fat, and polyunsaturated fat. Any solid fat is poor fat in general. Tropical oils like coconut and palm oil are also harmful. According to one rule of thumb, saturated and trans fats should account for no more than 10% of your daily calories. The calculation is simple since each gram of fat carries around 100 calories. If you consume 2,000 calories per day (the figure used as a guideline on nutrition labels), saturated and trans fats should account for no more than 200 calories. That's a limit of 20 grams of unhealthy fats each day. There are other dietary modifications you may make that can benefit you. Let's take a look at a few of them.

Chapter 4: Foods to include

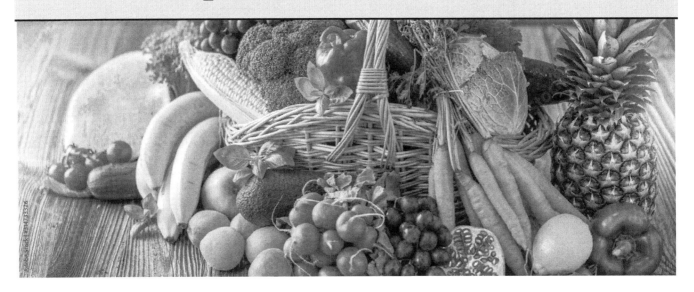

The Rainbow Rule

The basic guideline is to use as many colors as possible on your platter. You may be sure you're eating a well-balanced and healthy diet if your food contains the majority of the rainbow's color. Red foods, such as strawberries and red peppers; orange foods, such as carrots; yellow foods, such as corn and squash; green foods, such as kale and spinach; and blue foods, such as blueberries and grapes, should all be consumed in large amounts daily.

Fruit and vegetable consumption should be at least five to nine servings each day, with more being preferable. A serving isn't as big as you would imagine. One medium fruit or one cup raw small fruits, half a cup cooked vegetable, three-quarters cup juice, one cup leafy greens, or one cup raw vegetables. It's very simple to include veggies and fruits into meals. Make a spaghetti sauce with shredded carrots, banana bread, and fruit juice popsicles for your kids.

Eat More Fiber

Dietary fiber is divided into two types: soluble and insoluble fiber. Soluble fiber is important for lowering LDL cholesterol levels since it dissolves in water. It works by absorbing bile salts in the intestines. To make additional bile salts, the body removes cholesterol from the circulation. It's critical to consume 5 to 10 grams of soluble fiber every day. You may get this amount from your diet if you consume the 25 to 30 grams of dietary fiber suggested by the American Dietetic Association each day. Even more, fiber may be obtained by following a vegetarian diet. Fruits, vegetables, whole grains, and legumes are high in dietary fiber. Oat bran, strawberries, apples, citrus fruit, barley, beans, rice bran, and peas are high in soluble fiber. Most whole grains, carrots, cauliflower, apple peel, and beets include insoluble fiber, which may help you feel full and keep you regular but not affect cholesterol. Each serving of high-fiber food has at least 5 grams of fiber. An "excellent source" of fiber is defined as a food with more than 2.5 grams per serving.

Eat Healthy Fats

Doctors recognize that the optimal diet is high in healthy fats rather than one low in fat. Monounsaturated fats are the healthiest fats to consume. Extra-virgin olive oil, unrefined safflower oil, almonds, and avocados should all be included in your diet. Omega-3 fatty acids, which may be found in walnuts, tofu, soybeans, fatty fish, and flaxseed, are healthy fats to consume. Most Americans lack omega-3 fats and consume excessive omega-6 fats in polyunsaturated oils. The ratio of omega-3 to omega-6 is crucial for good health. This ratio may be improved by increasing monounsaturated fat intake.

Olive and Canola Oils

While you want to keep fat intake modest to maintain your ideal weight, oils like olive and canola may help decrease cholesterol levels. They are high in polyunsaturated fat, the healthiest kind of fat.

Fish

Omega-3 fatty acids are found in fish oils, and they help prevent blood vessel blockages and clots. According to medical experts, fish should be consumed at least twice a week.

Soy

Compounds in soy protein, such as those found in tofu, soybeans, and soy-based dairy substitutes, induce blood arteries to dilate efficiently, allowing the body to get the blood it needs. Antioxidants are also present, demonstrated to reduce the risk of cancer and heart disease.

Nuts

Nuts, like fish, are high in omega-3 fatty acids. However, since they are high in calories, you should have them in moderation.

Oats and Other Whole Grains

Several nutrients are present in oats and whole grains but are absent in refined grain products such as white flour. Oats also include water-soluble fiber, which studies have shown to decrease LDL cholesterol without reducing HDL cholesterol levels. Beans, barley, and wheat bran are other foods high in soluble fiber.

Chapter 5: Foods to avoid

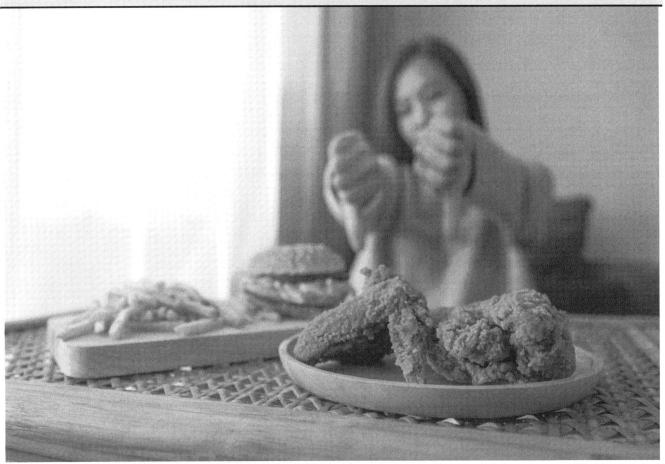

If you are trying to lower cholesterol and triglycerides, there are several things to avoid. Processed meats, fast foods and foods containing trans fats should be avoided. Also, reduce the number of sugary foods you eat and the amount of sugar in the dishes you currently eat. Most recipes can still be made with half to two-thirds of the specified sugar. Here are some details:

Saturated Fats

Saturated fats are the main reason for high cholesterol levels. Saturated fats, in general, are fats that are solid at room temperature. Saturated fats are classified into numerous categories, and the quantity of saturated fat in packaged goods in the United States is given on the nutrition information label. This implies you have complete control over how much-saturated fat you consume. According to the American Heart Association and others, you should consume no more than 20 grams of saturated fat each day. The recipes in this book will lead you to the cuts of meat and cooking procedures that will enable you to achieve your goal.

Red Meats

In terms of saturated fat, beef, pork, and lamb are often the worst. They indeed tend to have more than fish or poultry. However, the amount they have is highly dependent on the cut you choose. High-fat beef cuts might have up to five times the amount of saturated fat as lean cuts.

Poultry Skin

While poultry skin may not have as much saturated fat as red meat, it still has a substantial quantity. Compared to only the flesh, a chicken thigh with the skin contains almost 2 g more saturated fat. And in this instance, getting rid of the fat is simple—just don't eat the skin.

Whole-Milk Dairy

Dairy products are another category where making informed choices may lower saturated fat intake. Avoid full milk or cream-based products. Choose fat-free sour cream and cream cheese, as well as skim milk and reduced-fat cheeses. Instead of cream, use fat-free evaporated milk.

Tropical Oils

Saturated fats are present in some of the plant oils in this category. Palm, palm kernel, and coconut oils, as well as cocoa butter, are among them. Although they're normally simple to avoid, certain commercial baked products and processed meals may include them.

Trans Fats

Trans-fatty acids are another name for trans fats. They're made by combining hydrogen with vegetable oil in a process known as hydrogenation. The fat becomes more solid and less prone to deteriorate as a result. Trans fats are still a frequent component in commercially baked products and fried meals.

Trans fat content must be included on nutrition labels by food producers. The food label amounts less than 0.5 grams per serving, maybe 0-gram trans-fat.

Margarine and Other Hydrogenated Oils

Avoid hydrogenated or partly hydrogenated oils in margarine and solid shortening. Although some recipes in this book require margarine because the texture of the food requires it, liquid or soft margarine should be used whenever possible.

Commercial Baked Goods and Fried Foods

Read the labels on the products you buy and know that hydrogenated oils are popular in baked goods. Although public awareness has increased and many restaurants now cook in oils free of trans fats, be sure you know what you're consuming.

5.1 Useful and practical advice to improve health and lifestyle

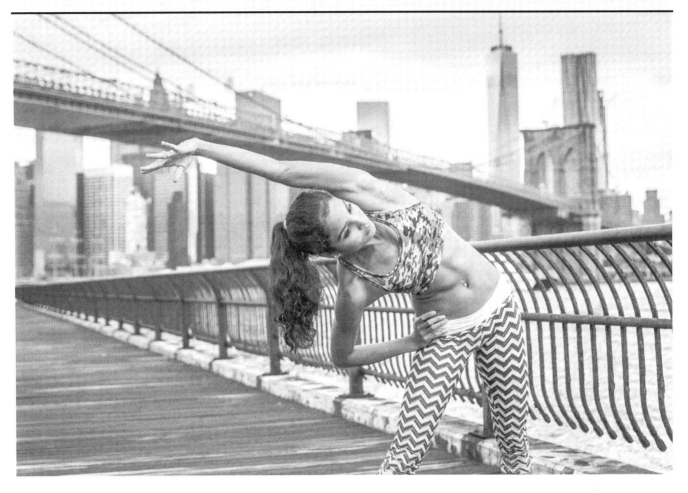

High cholesterol increases your risk of heart disease and heart attack. Medications may help you decrease your cholesterol levels. However, making certain lifestyle adjustments might be quite beneficial.

If you currently use drugs to decrease cholesterol, these changes may help them work better. Here they are:

1. **Eat heart-healthy foods**

A few dietary adjustments may help lower cholesterol and enhance heart health:

- Increase soluble fiber.
- Eliminate trans fats.
- Reduce saturated fats.
- Consume foods that are rich in omega-3 fatty acids.

- Add whey protein.

2. **Increase your physical activity by exercising most days of the week.**

3. **Quit smoking**

4. **Lose weight**

5. **Drink alcohol only in moderation**

Measuring Conversions

There are two widely employed measuring schemes in nutrition: Metric and US Customary.

Weight (mass)	
Metric (grams)	**US contemporary (ounces)**
14 grams	½ ounce
28 grams	1 ounce
85 grams	3 ounces
100 grams	3.53 ounces
113 grams	4 ounces
227 grams	8 ounces
340 grams	12 ounces
454 grams	16 ounces or 1 pound

Volume (liquid)

Metric	US Customary
.6 ml	⅛ tsp
1.2 ml	¼ tsp
2.5 ml	½ tsp
3.7 ml	¾ tsp
5 ml	1 tsp
15 ml	1 tbsp
30 ml	2 tbsp
59 ml	2 fluid ounces or ¼ cup
118 ml	½ cup
177 ml	¾ cup
237 ml	1 cup or 8 fluid ounces
1.9 liters	8 cups or ½ gallon

Oven Temperatures	
Metric	**US contemporary**
121° C	250° F
149° C	300° F
177° C	350° F
204° C	400° F
232° C	450° F

The table below shows normal lipogram ranges.

* High HDL cholesterols are desirable. It is the form cholesterol that removes it from the blood

	Normal	High	Very high
Total cholesterol	< 5.2 mmol/l	5.2-6.2 mmol/l	> 6.2 mmol/l
LDL-cholesterol	< 3.3 mmol/l	3.3 – 4.1 mmol/l	> 4.1 mmol/l
HDL-cholesterol	> 1 mmol/l	1.1 – 1.6 mmol/l*	> 1.6 mmol/l*
Triglycerides	< 1.7 mmol/l	1.7 – 2.3 mmol/l	> 2.3 mmol/l

Chapter 6: Breakfast Recipes

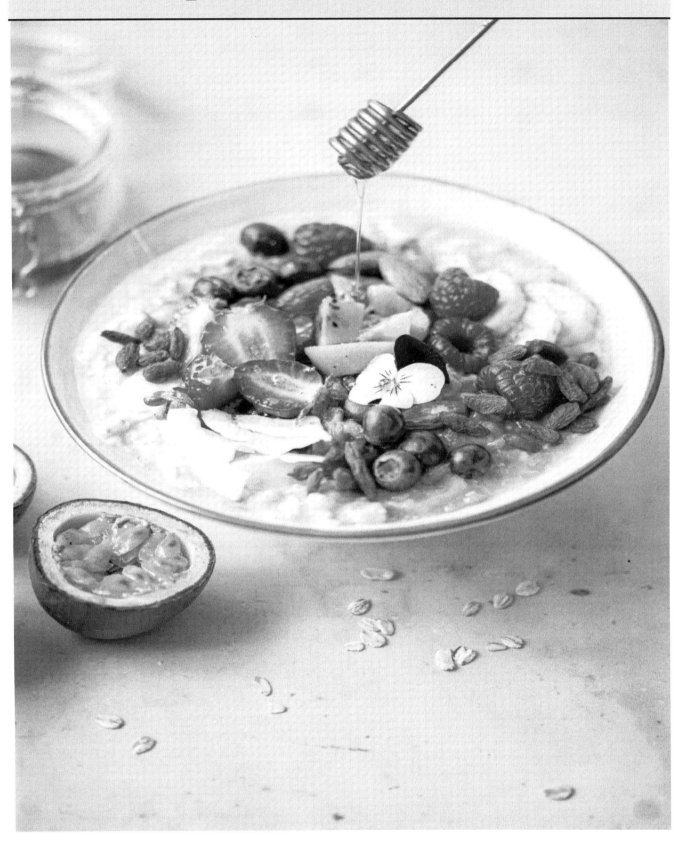

Berry Smoothie Bowl

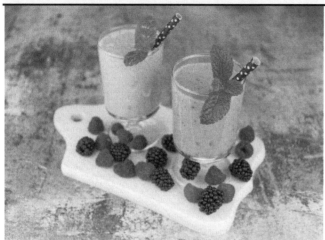

Preparation Time: 5 minutes/**Cooking Time:** 0 minutes/**Total Time:** 5 minutes

Servings: 2/**Difficulty Level:** Easy

Ingredients:

- 1 cup of fat-free milk
- 1 cup of frozen unsweetened strawberries
- 1/2 cup of frozen unsweetened raspberries
- 3 tablespoons of sugar
- 1 cup of ice cubes
- Optional: Sliced fresh strawberries, chia seeds, unsweetened shredded coconut, fresh raspberries, fresh pumpkin seeds, and sliced almonds

Instructions:

1. Combine the milk, berries, and sugar in a blender; cover and mix until smooth. Cover and process until smooth, adding ice cubes as needed.
2. To serve, divide the mixture into two serving dishes.
3. Optional toppings may be added as desired.

Nutritional Information: Calories: 155 kcal
Protein: 5 g | Carbohydrates: 35 g | Fat: 0 g
Cholesterol: 2 mg | Fiber: 2 g

Loaded Quinoa Breakfast Bowl

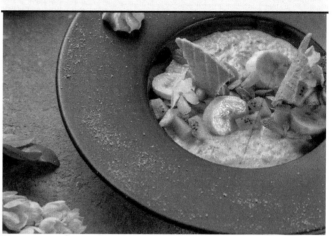

Preparation time: 15 minutes/**Cooking Time:** 15 minutes/**Total time:** 30 minutes

Servings: 1/**Difficulty Level:** Easy

Ingredients:

- 1/4 cup of tri-colored quinoa; rinsed
- 3/4 cup of water, divided
- 2 tablespoons of dried goji berries/ dried cranberries
- 1/4 cup of unsweetened almond milk
- 1 small banana
- 1/8 teaspoon of ground cinnamon
- 1 tablespoon of maple syrup
- 1/8 teaspoon of vanilla extract
- 1 tablespoon of chopped walnuts
- 1/4 cup of unsweetened fresh/frozen blueberries
- 1 tablespoon of slivered almonds
- Optional: More unsweetened almond milk & maple syrup
- 1 tablespoon of new pumpkin seeds

Instructions:
Bring 1/2 cup of water to a boil in a small saucepan. Stir in the quinoa. Reduce heat to low and cook, covered, for 12-15 minutes, or until liquid is absorbed. Meanwhile, soak the berries in the remaining water for about 10 minutes before draining. Bananas are halved crosswise; 1 banana half should be sliced, while the other should be mashed. Take the quinoa from the heat and fluff it with a fork. Add mashed banana, maple syrup, cinnamon, almond milk, and vanilla extract. After transferring to a separate bowl, add blueberries, pumpkin seeds, walnuts, banana slices, almonds, and goji berries. If

desired, top with extra almond milk and maple syrup.
Nutritional Information:
Calories: 475 kcal | protein: 13 g | carbohydrates: 83 g
| Fat: 13 g | Cholesterol: 0 mg | Fiber: 10 g

Overnight Peach Oatmeal

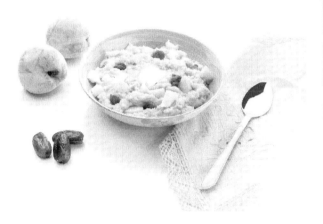

Preparation time: 10 minutes/**Cooking Time:** 7 hours/**Total time:** 7 hours 10 mines
Servings: 6/**Difficulty Level:** Medium
Ingredients:

- 1 cup of steel-cut oats
- 1/4 teaspoon of salt
- 4 cups of water
- 1/4 teaspoon of vanilla/ almond extract
- 3 tablespoons of brown sugar
- 1 cup of vanilla soy milk/ vanilla almond milk
- Optional toppings: brown sugar, cinnamon, sliced almonds, and additional peaches
- 2 medium peaches; sliced/ 3 cups of unsweetened frozen sliced peaches, thawed

Instructions:
Mix the first 6 ingredients in a well-greased 3-quart slow cooker. Cook on low for 7-8 hours, covered until oats are soft. Just before serving, add the peaches. Pressure cooker option: Reduce the amount of water to 3 cups. Pour into a 6-quart electric pressure cooker that has been sprayed with cooking spray. Add the soy milk, oats, salt, brown sugar, and vanilla. Close the pressure-release valve and lock the lid. Adjust to high pressure and cook for 4 minutes. Allow for a natural release of pressure. Just before serving, add the peaches. When the oatmeal rests for a while, it thickens. Optional toppings may be added if desired.
Nutritional Information:
Calories: 163 kcal, protein: 5 g, carbohydrates: 31 g, Fat: 2 g, Cholesterol: 0 mg, Fiber: 4 g

Pear-Stuffed French Vanilla Toast

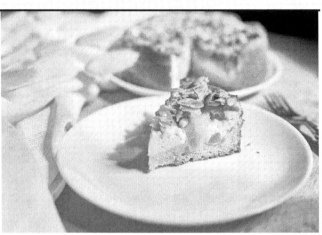

Preparation time: 30 minutes/**Cooking Time:** 40 minutes/**Total time:** 1 hour 10 mines/**Servings:** 6/**Difficulty Level:** Medium
Ingredients:

- 1/2 cup of butter, melted
- 1 cup of packed brown sugar
- 2 teaspoons of vanilla extract
- 1 large pear, peeled & sliced: (about 1-1/2 cups)
- 4 cups of cubed day-old French bread; (1-1/2-inch pieces)
- 3/4 cup of raisins
- 2 cups of French vanilla ice cream; melted
- 3/4 cup of finely chopped pecans
- 2 teaspoons of ground cinnamon
- 4 large eggs

Instructions:
Brown sugar & butter are combined in a small bowl. Spread the mixture on the bottom of an 8-inch square baking dish that has been buttered. Pears, bread cubes, raisins, and pecans are layered on top. Whisk together eggs, cinnamon, ice cream, and vanilla in a large mixing bowl until well combined; pour over top. Refrigerate for several hours or overnight, covered. Preheat the oven to 350 degrees Fahrenheit. While the oven warms up, remove the casserole from the refrigerator. Cook for 40-45 minutes, uncovered, or until golden brown and a knife inserted in the middle comes out clean.
Nutritional Information:
Calories: 701 kcal, protein: 15 g, carbohydrates: 80 g, Fat: 38 g, Cholesterol: 339 mg, Fiber: 4

Rise and Shine Parfait

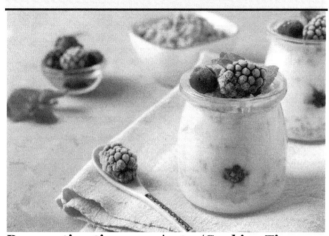

Preparation time: 15 minutes/**Cooking Time:** 0 minutes/**Total time:** 15 minutes
Servings: 4/**Difficulty Level:** Easy
Ingredients:
- 2 medium peaches; chopped
- 4 cups of fat-free vanilla yogurt
- 1/2 cup of granola without raisins / Lean Crunch cereal
- 2 cups of fresh blackberries

Instructions:
In 4 parfait glasses, layer half of the yogurt, blackberries, peaches, and granola. Layers are repeated.
Nutritional Information:
Calories: 259 kcal, protein: 13 g, carbohydrates: 48 g, Fat: 3 g, Cholesterol: 7 mg, Fiber: 7 g

Overnight Cherry-Almond Oatmeal

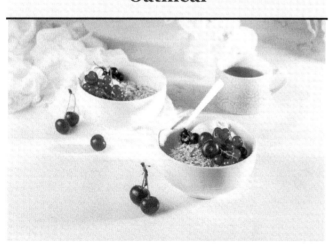

Preparation time: 10 minutes/**Cooking Time:** 7 hours/**Total time:** 7 hours 15 minutes/**Servings:** 6/**Difficulty Level:** Easy
Ingredients:
- 1 cup of steel-cut oats
- 4 cups of vanilla almond milk
- 1/3 cup of packed brown sugar
- 1 cup of dried cherries
- 1/2 teaspoon of salt
- Optional; Additional almond milk
- 1/2 teaspoon of ground cinnamon

Instructions:
Combine all ingredients in a 3-quart slow cooker covered with cooking spray. Cook on low for 7-8 hours, covered, until oats are soft. Before serving, give it a good stir. Serve with more milk if desired.
Nutritional Information:
Calories: 276 kcal, protein: 5 g, carbohydrates: 57 g, Fat: 4 g, Cholesterol: 0 mg, Fiber: 4 g

Banana Oatmeal Pancakes

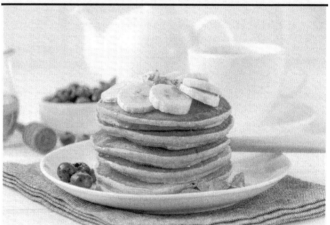

Preparation time: 10 minutes/**Cooking Time:** 5 min/**Total time:** 20 minutes
Servings: 8/**Difficulty Level:** Easy
Ingredients:
- 1 large firm banana; finely chopped
- 2 cups of complete whole wheat, pancake mix
- 1/4 cup of chopped walnuts
- 1/2 cup of old-fashioned oats

Instructions:
Follow the package instructions for making pancake batter. Add the oats, bananas, and walnuts. Pour 1/4 cupsful of batter onto a heated griddle covered with cooking spray; flip when bubbles appear on the surface. Cook till golden brown on the second side.
Nutritional Information:
Calories: 155 kcal, protein: 7 g, carbohydrates: 28 g, Fat: 4 g, Cholesterol: 0 mg, Fiber: 4 g

Garlic-Herb Mini Quiches

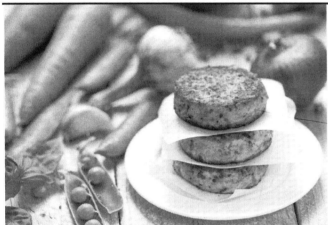

Preparation time: 25 minutes/**Cooking Time:** 0 minutes/**Total time:** 25 minutes
Servings: 45 Mini-Quiches/**Difficulty Level:** Medium
Ingredients:

- 1/4 cup of fat-free milk
- 1 package of (6-1/2 ounces) garlic-herb reduced-fat spreadable cheese
- 3 packages (1.9 ounces each) frozen miniature, phyllo tart shells
- 2 large eggs
- Minced chives, optional
- 2 tablespoons of minced fresh parsley

Instructions:
Preheat oven to 350°F. Beat the spreadable cheese, milk, and eggs in a small bowl. Fill each tart shell with 2 teaspoons of the mixture and place on an ungreased baking sheet. Serve with a parsley garnish. Bake for 10-12 minutes, or until the filling has set and the shells have browned somewhat. If desired, garnish with chives. Warm the dish before serving.

Nutritional Information:
Calories: 31 kcal, protein: 1 g, carbohydrates: 2 g, Fat: 2 g, Cholesterol: 12 mg, Fiber: 0 g

Oatmeal Waffles

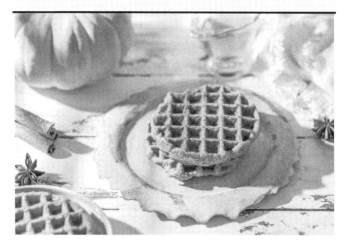

Preparation time: 25 minutes/**Cooking Time:** 10 minutes/**Total time:** 25 minutes
Servings: 10 waffles/**Difficulty Level:** Medium
Ingredients:

- 1/2 cup of whole wheat flour
- 1 cup of all-purpose flour
- 2 packets of instant maple & brown sugar/apple cinnamon oatmeal
- 1/4 teaspoon of salt
- 1 tablespoon of baking powder
- 1-1/2 cups of 2% milk
- 1 teaspoon of ground cinnamon
- 1/3 cup of butter; melted
- 2 eggs
- 1/2 cup of chopped pecans/walnuts

Instructions:
In a large mixing basin, combine the dry ingredients. In a separate bowl, whisk together the eggs, milk, and butter. Stir in the wet ingredients just until the dry ingredients are moistened. At this time, the pecans are folded in. In a preheated waffle iron, bake until golden brown, according to the manufacturer's instructions. Serve with a dollop of maple syrup on the side

Nutritional Information:
Calories: 205.9 kcal, protein: 10.4 g, carbohydrates: 30.0 g, Fat: 5.2 g, Cholesterol: 55.3 mg, Fiber: 4.3 g

Yogurt & Honey Fruit Cups

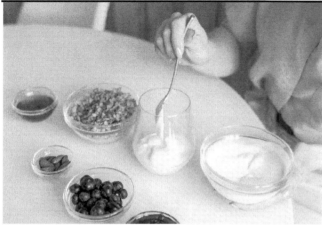

Preparation time: 10 minutes/**Cooking Time:** 0 minutes /**Total time:** 20 minutes
Servings: 6/**Difficulty Level:** Easy
Ingredients:
- 3/4 cup of vanilla, mandarin orange, or lemon yogurt
- 4-1/2 cups of cut-up fresh fruit (apples, pears, grapes, bananas, etc.)
- 1 tablespoon of honey
- 1/4 teaspoon of almond extract
- 1/2 teaspoon of grated orange zest

Instructions:
Fruit should be divided into 6 separate serving bowls. Toss the fruit with the orange zest, yogurt, honey, and extract.
Nutritional Information:
Calories: 97 kcal, protein: 2 g, carbohydrates: 23 g, Fat: 0 g, Cholesterol: 2 mg, Fiber: 2 g

Chicken and Asparagus Crepes

Preparation time: 1 hour plus chilling time/**Cooking Time:** 20 minutes /**Total time:** 1 hour 30 minutes/**Servings:** 12/**Difficulty Level:** Medium
Ingredients:
- 2 tablespoons of butter, melted
- 3 eggs
- 1-1/2 cups of 2% milk
- 1/4 teaspoon of salt
- 1 cup of all-purpose flour
- filling:
- 1 teaspoon of canola oil
- 1-1/2 cups of cut fresh asparagus; (1-inch pieces)
- 1 small onion; chopped
- 3 cups of cubed rotisserie chicken
- 2-1/2 cups of sliced fresh mushrooms

sauce:
- 1/8 teaspoon of pepper
- 1/4 teaspoon of salt
- 1-1/2 cups of 2% milk
- 1/4 cup of all-purpose flour
- 2/3 cup of part-skim shredded mozzarella cheese
- 1/4 cup of butter, cubed
- 6 slices of Swiss cheese, halved

Instructions:
Whisk the milk, eggs, and butter in a large mixing bowl. Combine the flour & salt; add to the egg mixture and combine well. Refrigerate it for 1 hour. Over medium heat, gently butter an 8-inch nonstick pan and pour 1/4 cup batter into the middle. Lift and tilt the pan to evenly coat the bottom. Cook until the top seems dry, then flip and cook for another 15-20 seconds. Place on a wire rack to cool. Continue with the remaining batter, re-greasing the skillet as necessary. When the crepes are cold, layer them with waxed paper/ paper towels between them. In a skillet, sauté the asparagus and onion until they are soft. Cook for another 2 minutes after adding the mushrooms. Remove the pan from the heat and add the chicken. Set it aside.
Melt the butter in a small pot over medium heat for the sauce. Stir in the salt, flour, and pepper until smooth, then add the milk in a slow, steady stream. Bring to a boil, then reduce to low heat and simmer, constantly stirring, for 2 minutes, or until the sauce has thickened.
Fill each crepe halfway with filling, then top with the two tablespoons sauce and 1 slice of Swiss cheese. Roll up and lay in two greased 11x7-inch baking trays, seam side down. Cheese mozzarellas are sprinkled on top. Bake for 20-25 minutes, uncovered, at 350° F, or until bubbling.
Nutritional Information:
Calories: 394.9 kcal, protein: 22.3 g, carbohydrates: 17.6 g, Fat: 23.1 g, Cholesterol: 140 mg, Fiber: 2 g

Banana Oat Breakfast Cookies

Preparation time: 20 minutes/**Cooking Time:** 15 minutes/bake /**Total time:** 50 minutes/**Servings:** 1 dozen/**Difficulty Level:** Medium
Ingredients:
- 1/2 cup of chunky peanut butter
- 1 cup of mashed ripe bananas; (about 2 medium)
- 1/2 cup of honey
- 1 cup of old-fashioned oats
- 1 teaspoon of vanilla extract

- 1/4 cup of nonfat dry milk powder
- 1/2 cup of whole wheat flour
- 1/2 teaspoon of salt
- 2 teaspoons of ground cinnamon
- 1 cup of dried cranberries/ raisins
- 1/4 teaspoon of baking soda

Instructions:
Preheat the oven to 350 degrees Fahrenheit. Blend bananas, honey, peanut butter, and vanilla in a mixing bowl until smooth. In a separate dish, whisk together dry ingredients; gradually fold into the wet mixture. Add the dried cranberries and mix well. Drop the dough by 1/4 cupsful onto prepared baking sheets, 3 inches apart, and flatten to 1/2-inch thickness.
Bake for 14-16 minutes, or until golden brown. Allow 5 minutes for cooling on the pans. Place on wire racks to cool. Serve warm or serve it at room temperature is OK. Microwave the cookie on high for 15-20 seconds or until warmed to reheat enough.

Nutritional Information:
Calories: 212 kcal, protein: 5 g, carbohydrates: 38 g, Fat: 6 g, Cholesterol: 38 mg, Fiber: 4 g

Zucchini Tomato Frittata

Preparation time: 20 minutes/**Cooking Time:** 15 minutes /**Total time:** 35 minutes
Servings: 4/**Difficulty Level:** Medium
Ingredients:
- 1 cup of boiling water
- 1/3 cup of sun-dried tomatoes; (not packed in oil)
- 1-1/2 cups of egg substitute
- 2 green onions; chopped
- 2 teaspoons of canola oil
- 1/2 cup of 2% cottage cheese
- 1/4 cup of minced fresh basil/1 tablespoon of dried basil
- 2 tablespoons of grated Parmesan cheese
- 1 cup of sliced zucchini
- 1/8 teaspoon of crushed red pepper flakes
- 1 medium sweet red pepper; chopped
- 1 cup of fresh broccoli florets

Instructions:
In a small dish, place the tomatoes. Allow 5 minutes after covering with boiling water. Drain the water and put it aside. Set aside the cottage cheese, egg substitute, onions, pepper flakes, basil, and saved tomatoes in a large mixing bowl. Sauté the broccoli, zucchini, and red pepper in oil in a 10-inch ovenproof

pan until soft. Reduce the heat to low and top with the reserved egg mixture. Cook, covered, for 4-6 minutes, or until almost set. Remove the lid from the skillet. Parmesan cheese is sprinkled on top. Broil for 2-3 minutes, or until eggs are set, at 3-4 inches from the flame. Allow for a 5-minute rest period. Cut the wedges in half.
Nutritional Information:
Calories: 138 kcal, protein: 15 g, carbohydrates: 11 g, Fat: 4 g, Cholesterol: 6 mg, Fiber: 3 g

Apple Pancakes

Preparation time: 20 minutes/**Cooking Time:** 0 minutes /**Total time:** 20 minutes
Servings: 10/**Difficulty Level:** Medium
Ingredients:
- Sugar substitute that is equivalent to 2 tsp sugar
- 2 cups of reduced-fat biscuit/baking mix
- 1 teaspoon of baking powder
- 1/4 teaspoon of salt
- 1 teaspoon of ground cinnamon
- 1 cup of fat-free milk
- 1/4 cup of egg substitute
- 1 tart apple; peeled & grated
- 2 teaspoons of vanilla extract

Instructions:
Combine the sugar substitute, biscuit mix, cinnamon, baking powder, and salt in a large mixing bowl. Combine the milk, egg substitute, and vanilla in a small dish; mix into the dry ingredients. Add the apple and fold it's in. Pour 1/4 cupsful of batter onto a heated pan sprayed with cooking spray; flip when bubbles appear on the surface. Cook till golden brown on the second side.
Nutritional Information:
Calories: 117 kcal, protein: 3 g, carbohydrates: 21 g, Fat: 2 g, Cholesterol: 1 mg, Fiber: 0 g

Breakfast Banana Splits

Preparation time: 10 minutes/**Cooking Time:** 0 minutes /**Total time:** 10 minutes
Servings: 2/**Difficulty Level:** Easy
Ingredients:
- 1/3 cup of each fresh blueberry, sliced peeled kiwifruit, halved seedless grapes and halved fresh strawberries
- 1 medium banana
- 1 cup of vanilla yogurt
- 2 maraschino cherries with stems
- 1/2 cup of granola with fruit & nuts

Instructions:
Bananas are cut in half crosswise. Split each banana in half lengthwise and arrange banana splits covered with remaining ingredients in a serving dish for each serving.

Nutritional Information:
Calories: 337 kcal, protein: 12 g, carbohydrates: 66 g, Fat: 6 g, Cholesterol: 6 mg, Fiber: 8 g

Pumpkin Pie Oatmeal

Preparation time: 15 minutes/**Cooking Time:** 0 minutes/**Total time:** 15 minutes
Servings: 2/**Difficulty Level:** Easy
Ingredients:
- 1/4 teaspoon of pumpkin pie spice
- 1/2 cup of canned pumpkin
- 1 cup of old-fashioned oats
- 2 tablespoons of sugar
- 1 cup of vanilla soy milk
- Optional: Dried cranberries & salted pumpkin seeds/petites
- 1 cup of water
- 1/4 teaspoon of vanilla extract

Instructions:
Combine the milk, pumpkin, oats, and pie spice in a small saucepan. Bring to a boil, then reduce to low heat and simmer for 5 minutes, stirring occasionally. Remove the pan from the heat and mix in the sugar and vanilla extract. If preferred, sprinkle cranberries & pumpkin seeds, then drizzle with more milk.

Nutritional Information:
Calories: 268 kcal, protein: 10 g, carbohydrates: 49 g, Fat: 5 g, Cholesterol: 0 mg, Fiber: 6 g

Autumn Power Porridge

Preparation time: 15 minutes/**Cooking Time:** 30 minutes/**Total time:** 45 minutes
Servings: 4/**Difficulty Level:** Easy
Ingredients:
- 3/4 cup of steel-cut oats
- 3 cups of water
- 1/4 teaspoon of salt
- 1/2 cup of quinoa, rinsed
- 3/4 cup of canned pumpkin
- 3 tablespoons of agave nectar/ maple syrup
- 1 teaspoon of pumpkin pie spice
- 1/2 cup of dried cranberries
- Milk; optional
- 1/3 cup of coarsely chopped walnuts; toasted

Instructions:
Combine the water, quinoa, oats, and salt in a large saucepan. Bring the water to a boil. Reduce the heat to low, cover, and cook for 20 minutes.
Combine the pie spice, pumpkin, and agave nectar in a mixing bowl. Remove from the heat, cover, and set aside for 5 minutes, or until the water has been absorbed and the grains have become soft. Add cranberries and walnuts to a mixing bowl. If preferred, serve with milk.

Nutritional Information:
Calories: 361 kcal, protein: 9 g, carbohydrates: 65 g, Fat: 10 g, Cholesterol: 0 mg, Fiber: 7 g

Brunch-Style Portobello Mushrooms

Preparation time: 10 minutes/**Cooking Time:** 20 minutes/**Total time:** 30 minutes
Servings: 4/**Difficulty Level:** Medium
Ingredients:
- 4 large Portobello mushrooms; stems removed
- 2 packages of frozen creamed spinach, thawed (10 ounces each)
- 4 large eggs
- 1/4 cup of shredded Gouda cheese
- 1/2 cup of crumbled cooked bacon
- Salt & pepper; optional

Instructions:
Place the mushrooms, stem side up, in a 15x10x1-inch baking pan that hasn't been buttered. Build up the sides of the mushrooms with spinach. Crack an egg carefully into the middle of each mushroom, then top with bacon and cheese. Preheat oven to 375°F and bake for 18-20 minutes, or until eggs are set. If desired, season with salt and pepper.

Nutritional Information:
Calories: 168 kcal, protein: 12 g, carbohydrates: 4 g, Fat: 11 g, Cholesterol: 108 mg, Fiber: 1 g

Pear-Blueberry Granola

Preparation time: 15 minutes/**Cooking Time:** 3 hours/**Total time:** 3 hours 20 minutes/**Servings:** 10/**Difficulty Level:** Medium
Ingredients:
- 2 cups of fresh/frozen unsweetened blueberries
- 5 medium pears, peeled & thinly sliced
- 1/2 cup of packed brown sugar
- 1 tablespoon of all-purpose flour

- 1/3 cup of apple cider/ unsweetened apple juice
- 2 tablespoons of butter
- 1 tablespoon of lemon juice
- 3 cups of granola without raisins
- 2 teaspoons of ground cinnamon

Instructions:
Combine all ingredients in a 4-quart slow cooker except granola and butter. Make a butter smear. Granola is sprinkled on top. Cook for 3-4 hours on low, or until fruit is soft.

Nutritional Information:
Calories: 267 kcal, protein: 7 g, carbohydrates: 51 g, Fat: 7 g, Cholesterol: 6 mg, Fiber: 10 g

Bagel Avocado Toast

Preparation time: 5 minutes/**Cooking Time:** 5 minutes/**Total time:** 10 minutes
Servings: 1/**Difficulty Level:** Easy
Ingredients:
- 1 slice of whole-grain bread; toasted
- ¼ medium avocado; mashed
- Pinch of flaky sea salt (Malden)
- 2 teaspoons of everything bagel seasoning

Instructions:
Avocados are spread on toast. Season it with salt and pepper.

Nutritional Information:
Calories: 172 kcal, protein: 5.4 g, carbohydrates: 17.8 g, Fat: 9.8 g, Cholesterol: 2 mg, Fiber: 5.9 g

Tropical Yogurt

Preparation time: 5 minutes/**Cooking Time:**/**Total time:** 5 minutes
Servings: 4/**Difficulty Level:** Easy
Ingredients:
- 1 can of (8 ounces) crushed unsweetened pineapple; drained
- 1/4 teaspoon of grated lime zest
- 2 cups of reduced-fat plain yogurt
- 1/4 teaspoon of coconut extract
- 2 teaspoons of sugar

Instructions:
Combine all ingredients in a small bowl. Chill until ready to serve.

Nutritional Information:
Calories: 121 kcal, protein: 7 g, carbohydrates: 20 g, Fat: 2 g, Cholesterol: 7 mg, Fiber: 0 g

Smoked Salmon Breakfast Wraps

Preparation time: minutes/**Cooking Time:** 0 minutes/**Total time:** 20 minutes
Servings: 4/**Difficulty Level:** Easy
Ingredients:
- 1 tablespoon of snipped fresh chives
- □ cup of light cream cheese spread
- 1 teaspoon of lemon peel; finely shredded
- 4 6 to 7-inch of whole wheat flour tortillas
- 1 tablespoon of lemon juice
- 3 ounces of smoked salmon (lox-style); thinly sliced, cut into strips
- 4 Lemon wedges
- 1 small zucchini; trimmed

Instructions:
Cream together chives, lemon peel, cream cheese, and lemon juice in a small bowl until creamy. Leave a 1/2-inch border around the edges of the tortillas after spreading evenly.
Distribute the salmon among the tortillas, putting it on the bottom half of each. To make zucchini ribbons, use a sharp vegetable peeler to cut extremely thin slices lengthwise along the zucchini. Serve the fish with zucchini ribbons on top. Tortillas should be rolled up from the bottom up. Slice in half. Serve with lemon wedges if preferred.

Nutritional Information:
Calories: 124 kcal, protein: 11.5 g, carbohydrates: 14.4 g, Fat: 6 g, Cholesterol: 14.8 mg, Fiber: 8.6 g

Mixed-Grain Muesli

Preparation time: 30 minutes/**Cooking Time:** 20 minutes /**Total time:** 12 hours 30 minutes/**Servings:** 4/**Difficulty Level:** Medium
Ingredients:
- 3 tablespoons of steel-cut oats
- 1 ¼ cups of water
- 3 tablespoons of quick-cooking barley
- 1 tablespoon of honey
- 3 tablespoons of cracked wheat
- ½ cup of fat-free milk
- ⅛ teaspoon of salt
- ¼ teaspoon of apple pie spice /pumpkin pie spice
- 1 small red-skin apple; cored and chopped
- ¼ cup of coarsely chopped pecans, almonds, or walnuts, toasted
- 3 tablespoons of assorted dried fruit (such as blueberries, snipped plums cranberries, snipped apricots, and dried fruit bits)

Instructions:

Combine the oats, barley, water, and cracked wheat in a 2-quart saucepan. Bring to a boil, then turn off the heat. Simmer for 8 minutes, uncovered. Cool for 5 minutes in a medium mixing bowl. Add milk, yogurt, apple pie spice, honey, and salt. Refrigerate for at least 12 hours or up to 3 days after covering. Transfer the cereal to a medium saucepan to serve. Cook, constantly stirring, over low heat until well heated. Divide the mixture into serving dishes. Add dried fruit and apple. Almonds are sprinkled on top. Tips: It's also possible to eat the cereal cold. Allow 15 minutes for it to come to room temperature before serving. To toast entire nuts or big chunks, lay them on parchment paper in a shallow baking pan. Bake for 5 to 10 minutes, or until brown, at 350 degrees F, shaking pan once or twice.

Nutritional Information:

Calories: 203 kcal, protein: 7.4 g, carbohydrates: 36.4 g, Fat: 4.3 g, Cholesterol: 3.2 mg, Fiber: 4.8 g

Breakfast Parfaits

Preparation time: 10 minutes/**Cooking Time:** 0 minutes/**Total time:** 10 minutes
Servings: 4/**Difficulty Level:** Easy
Ingredients:
- 1 cup of fresh/frozen raspberries
- 2 cups of pineapple chunks
- 1 cup of vanilla yogurt
- 1/2 cup of chopped dates or raisins
- 1/4 cup of sliced almonds
- 1 cup of sliced ripe banana

Instructions:

Layer the yogurt, dates, raspberries, pineapple, and banana in 4 parfait glasses or serving plates. Almonds are sprinkled on top. Serve right away.

Nutritional Information:

Calories: 277 kcal, protein: 5 g, carbohydrates: 60 g, Fat: 4 g, Cholesterol: 3 mg, Fiber: 6 g

Blueberry Muffins

Preparation time: 15 minutes/**Cooking Time:** 25 minutes/**Total time:** 1 hour
Servings: 12/**Difficulty Level:** Easy
Ingredients:
- ¼ cup of coconut flour
- 1 ¾ cups of almond flour
- ¼ teaspoon of baking soda
- 1 tablespoon of baking powder
- 1 cup of blueberries
- 1 ½ teaspoon of vanilla extract
- ¼ teaspoon of salt

- ½ cup of reduced-fat milk
- 3 large eggs
- ¼ cup of avocado oil
- ☐ cup and 2 tablespoons of light brown sugar

Instructions:

Preheat an oven to 350 degrees Fahrenheit. Using cooking spray, generously coat a muffin tray. Sift together coconut flour, baking soda, almond flour, baking powder, and salt in a large mixing bowl. Toss in the blueberries to coat. Whisk the brown sugar, eggs, oil, milk, and vanilla extract in a medium mixing bowl. Stir in the wet ingredients until well blended. Using roughly 1/4 cup batter per muffin cup, divide batter among muffin cups.
Bake the muffins for 20 to 25 minutes, or until it turns light brown around the edges and the toothpick inserted in the middle comes out clean. Allow it cool for 20 minutes in a pan on a wire rack. Remove it from tin and cool thoroughly.

Nutritional Information:

Calories: 204 kcal, protein: 5.8 g, carbohydrates: 14.9 g, Fat: 14.6 g, Cholesterol: 47.3 mg, Fiber: 2.9 g

Cinnamon Streusel Rolls

Preparation time: 45 minutes/**Cooking Time:** 30 minutes/**Total time:** 2 hours 45 minutes/**Servings:** 15/**Difficulty Level:** Hard
Ingredients:
- 2 teaspoons of packed brown sugar
- ¼ teaspoon of vanilla extract
- 1 cup of fat-free milk and 2 to 3 teaspoons; divided
- ¼ cup of tub-style; 60-70% vegetable oil spread; divided
- ¼ cup of warm water (110 to 115 degrees F)
- 1 teaspoon of salt
- 4-4 1/2 cups of all-purpose flour
- ¼ cup of powdered sugar
- 1 package of active dry yeast
- ½ cup of rolled oats; toasted
- ¼ cup of refrigerated/frozen egg product; thawed/ 1 egg; lightly beaten
- 2 teaspoons of ground cinnamon
- ☐ cup of light sour cream
- ¼ cup of chopped pecans; toasted

Instructions:

In a small saucepan, heat and whisk 1 cup of milk, 2 tablespoons of vegetable oil spread, brown sugar, and salt just until heated (110 to 115 degrees F); leave aside. In a large mixing bowl, combine the warm water & yeast; set aside for 10 minutes. Toss the yeast mixture with the egg and milk mixture. With a wooden spoon, stir in the flour substitute and as much of the leftover all-purpose flour as you can. On a lightly floured surface, roll out the dough. Knead in enough residual flour to form a soft, smooth, and elastic dough (3 to 5 minutes total). Form a ball out of the dough. Turn once to coat the surface and place in a lightly oiled bowl. Allow rising until doubled in size in a warm location (about 1 hour). Punch the dough down. Turn the dough out onto a floured board. Cover and set aside for 10 minutes to allow flavors to meld.

Meanwhile, carefully oil and put aside a 13x9-inch baking pan. In a medium mixing bowl, combine the oats and cinnamon. Blend in the remaining 2 tablespoons of vegetable oil distributed with your fingertips until the mixture is crumbly. Add the pecans and mix well.

Make a 15x8-inch rectangle out of the dough. Sprinkle the pecan mixture over one of the long sides, leaving a 1-inch gap. Begin rolling up the long side with the topping in a spiral. Pinch the seam of the dough to seal it, then cut it into 15 equal pieces. Arrange the pieces in a prepared baking pan cut sides up. Allow rising until almost doubled in size in a warm place (about 30 minutes).

Preheat the oven to 375 degrees Fahrenheit and bake for 25–30 minutes, or until golden brown. Cool for 5 minutes in the pan on a wire rack. Meanwhile, whisk together the sour cream, vanilla, powdered sugar, and 2 to 3 tablespoons of milk to make a drizzling consistency. Take the rolls out of the pan. Drizzle frosting on top. Warm the dish before serving

Nutritional Information:
Calories: 194 kcal, protein: 5.2 g, carbohydrates: 32.5 g, Fat: 4.8 g, Cholesterol: 1.8 mg, Fiber: 3.3 g

Apple Cinnamon Chia Pudding

Preparation time: 10 minutes/**Cooking Time:** 0 minutes/**Total time:** 8 hours 10 minutes/**Servings:** 1/**Difficulty Level:** Hard
Ingredients:
- 2 tablespoons of chia seeds
- ½ cup of unsweetened almond milk / other nondairy milk
- ¼ teaspoon of vanilla extract
- 2 teaspoons of pure maple syrup
- ¼ teaspoon of ground cinnamon
- 1 tablespoon of chopped toasted pecans; divided
- ½ cup of diced apple; divided

Instructions:
Combine chia, vanilla, almond milk (non-dairy milk), maple syrup, and cinnamon in a small bowl.

Refrigerate for approximately 8 hours and for up to 3 days after covering. When ready for serving, give it a good stir. Half of the pudding should be spooned into a serving glass (or bowl), followed by half of the apple and pecans. Top with remaining apple & pecans and the remainder of the pudding.

Nutritional Information:
Calories: 233 kcal, protein: 4.8 g, carbohydrates: 27.7 g, Fat: 12.7 g, Cholesterol: 1 mg, Fiber: 10.1 g

Watermelon and Berry salad with buckwheat

Preparation time: 10 minutes/**Cooking Time:** 5 minutes /**Total time:** 15 minutes
Servings: 4/**Difficulty Level:** Easy
Ingredients:
- 800g seedless watermelon; skin removed; cut into wedges
- 2 tbsp. of pistachios; coarsely chopped
- 250g strawberries; hulled, halved
- 2 tbsp. of shredded coconut
- 2/3 cup of natural yogurt; to serve
- 2 tbsp. of raw buckwheat kernels
- 125g fresh raspberries

Instructions:
Preheat the oven to 180 degrees Celsius/160 degrees' Celsius fan-forced. Using the baking paper, line a baking pan. In a mixing dish, combine the coconut, buckwheat, and pistachios. Spread buckwheat mixture evenly over the prepared baking pan and bake for 5 minutes, stirring once, or until light brown.On serving plates, arrange the strawberry, watermelon, and raspberries. Top each with a dollop of yogurt and a sprinkle of the buckwheat mixture.

Nutritional Information:
Calories: 189 kcal, protein: 7 g, carbohydrates: 22 g, Fat: 7 g, Cholesterol: 1 mg, Fiber: 5 g

Healthy Breakfast Muffins

Preparation time: 10 minutes/**Cooking Time:** 20 minutes /**Total time:** 30 minutes
Servings: 6/**Difficulty Level:** Easy
Ingredients:
- 1/2 cup of moist coconut flakes
- 3/4 cup of whole meal flour
- 1/2 cup of coconut sugar
- 3/4 cup of plain flour
- 1/2 cup of milk
- 2 tsp of baking powder
- 1/3 cup of light olive oil

- 1/2 cup of Fruit and Chia Spread Mango; Passionfruit & Chia Seeds; warmed
- 1 egg; lightly whisked

Instructions:
Preheat the oven to 180°F/160°F fan force. Paper cases should be used to line six 200ml muffin holes. Whisk together the coconut sugar, coconut flakes, flours, and baking powder using a whisk. In the middle, dig a well. Add oil, milk, and egg. Mix everything with a large metal spoon until it's just blended. Add the jam and mix well.
Fill muffin tins halfway with the mixture. Bake for 15-18 minutes, or until a skewer inserted in the middle comes out clean on one of the muffins. Allow cooling before serving. Brush with passionfruit, warmed mango, and chia jam, if desired.

Nutritional Information:
Calories: 175 kcal, protein: 4.5 g, carbohydrates: 24 g, Fat: 7 g, Cholesterol: 32 mg, Fiber: 2.1 g

Turkey Breakfast Sausage

Preparation time: 10 minutes/**Cooking Time:** 10 minutes /**Total time:** 20 minutes
Servings: 8/**Difficulty Level:** Easy
Ingredients:
- 1/4 teaspoon of black pepper
- 1-pound ground turkey
- 3/4 teaspoon of dried sage
- 1/4 teaspoon of white pepper
- 1/2 teaspoon of garlic powder
- 1/4 teaspoon of ground mace
- 1/4 teaspoon of onion powder
- 1 teaspoon of olive oil
- 1/4 teaspoon of ground allspice

Instructions:
Mix all the ingredients well. Preheat oven to 325°F and fry, grill, or bake on a prepared baking sheet until desired doneness or 10 minutes.
Nutritional Information:
Calories: 69 kcal, protein: 13 g, carbohydrates: 1 g, Fat: 7 g, Cholesterol: 41 mg, Fiber: 0 g

Vegetable Omelet

Preparation time: 5 minutes/**Cooking Time:** 5 minutes /**Total time:** 10 minutes
Servings: 2/**Difficulty Level:** Easy
Ingredients:

- 1/4 cup of onion; diced
- 1 tablespoon of olive oil
- 1/4 cup of green bell peppers; diced
- 2 ounces' mushrooms; sliced
- 1/4 cup of zucchini; sliced
- 2 tablespoons of fat-free sour cream
- 1/2 cup of tomato; diced
- 2 ounces' Swiss cheese; shredded
- 1 cup of egg substitute
- 2 tablespoons of water

Instructions:
In a large pan, heat the olive oil and cook the mushrooms, zucchini, green bell pepper, onion, and tomato until tender, finishing with the tomato. Combine the sour cream egg substitute, and whisk until frothy. Place an omelet pan or skillet over medium-high heat and coat with the nonstick veggie spray. Fill the pan with the egg mixture. As it cooks, lift the sides to enable the raw egg to flow below. Cover half of the eggs with cheese and sautéed veggies when almost set, then fold another half over. Cook the eggs until they are set.
Nutritional Information:
Calories: 263 kcal, protein: 25 g, carbohydrates: 8 g, Fat: 13 g, Cholesterol: 17 mg, Fiber: 2 g

Breakfast Potatoes

Preparation time: 5 minutes/**Cooking Time:** 15 minutes /**Total time:** 20 minutes
Servings: 6/**Difficulty Level:** Easy
Ingredients:
- 1/4 cup of green bell peppers; chopped
- 1 cup of onion; chopped
- 4 potatoes
- 1/2 teaspoon of freshly ground black pepper
- 1 tablespoon of unsalted margarine

Instructions:
Potatoes are boiled or microwaved until nearly done. Drain them and, coarsely, chop them and combine them with onion & green bell pepper. In a wide skillet, melt margarine. Toss in the potato mixture. Add a pinch of black pepper to the top. Fry till golden brown, flipping often.
Nutritional Information:
Calories: 201 kcal, protein: 5 g, carbohydrates: 42 g, Fat: 2 g, Cholesterol: 0 mg, Fiber: 5 g

Couscous Cereal with Fruit

Preparation time: 5 minutes/**Cooking Time:** 5 minutes /**Total time:** 10 minutes
Servings: 2/**Difficulty Level:** Easy

Ingredients:

- 2 tablespoons of raisins
- 1/2 cup of couscous
- 3/4 cup of water
- 2 tablespoons of dried cranberries
- 1/2 teaspoon of cinnamon
- 1 tablespoon of honey

Instructions:

Bring a pot of water to a gentle boil. Stir in the couscous, then cover & remove from the heat. Allow for a 5-minute rest period. Add the remaining ingredients.

Nutritional Information:

Calories: 250 kcal, protein: 6 g, carbohydrates: 57 g, Fat: 2 g, Cholesterol: 0 mg, Fiber: 3 g

French Toast

Preparation time: 5 minutes/**Cooking Time:** 15 minutes /**Total time:** 20 minutes
Servings: 4/**Difficulty Level:** Easy
Ingredients:

- 3/4 cup of skim milk
- 1/2 cup of egg substitute
- 2 teaspoons of vanilla extract
- 8 slices of day-old, whole wheat bread
- 1/2 teaspoon of cinnamon

Instructions:

Whisk the egg substitute, vanilla, milk, and cinnamon in a large mixing bowl or dish. Dip both sides of the bread into the egg mixture. Place a griddle or nonstick skillet over medium-high heat and coat with the nonstick vegetable oil spray. Cook for at least 3 minutes on each side, or until both sides of bread are golden brown, on a pan or skillet.

Nutritional Information:

Calories: 185 kcal, protein: 11 g, carbohydrates: 27 g, Fat: 3 g, Cholesterol: 1 mg, Fiber: 2 g

Pasta Frittata

Preparation time: 10 minutes/**Cooking Time:** 20 minutes /**Total time:** 30 minutes
Servings: 4/**Difficulty Level:** Medium
Ingredients:

- 1 cup of onion; chopped
- 2 tablespoons of olive oil
- 1 cup of red bell pepper; diced
- 2 cups of cooked pasta
- 1 cup of egg substitute
- 1/4 cup of grated Parmesan

Instructions:

Preheat a broiler-safe nonstick skillet with a 1 Q-inch (25-cm) diameter. When the pan is heated, add the oil, and cook the red bell pepper and onion, stirring regularly, for 2 to 3 minutes. Toss the pasta into the pan and toss thoroughly. Flatten the pasta onto the pan's bottom using a spatula when all the ingredients are fully mixed. Allow it to simmer for a few more minutes. Whisk the egg substitute and the grated Parmesan cheese in a separate bowl. Pour the egg mixture over pasta, ensuring eggs are equally distributed. Lift the edges of the pasta gently to allow the egg to pour beneath and coat the pasta fully. Allow 6 to 9 minutes for the eggs to cook. Finish cooking by placing the pan on the hot broiler.

Nutritional Information:

Calories: 360 kcal, protein: 18 g, carbohydrates: 46 g, Fat: 12 g, Cholesterol: 6 mg, Fiber: 3 g

Breakfast Quesadilla

Preparation time: 5 minutes/**Cooking Time:** 10 minutes /**Total time:** 15 minutes
Servings: 4/**Difficulty Level:** Medium
Ingredients:

- 1 cup of egg substitute
- 1/4 cup of salsa
- 1/4 cup of low-fat cheddar cheese; shredded
- 8 corn tortillas

Instructions:

Prepare the scrambled eggs, using egg replacer and when almost ready, mix in the salsa and cheese. Using a nonstick olive oil spray, lightly coat one side of the tortillas and arrange four of them oiled side down on a baking sheet. Spread the egg mixture among the tortillas, smoothing it evenly. The remaining tortillas, oiled side up, go on top. Grill the quesadillas for 3 minutes on each side, or until golden brown. To serve, cut into quarters.

Nutritional Information:

Calories: 152 kcal, protein: 12 g, carbohydrates: 18 g, Fat: 4 g, Cholesterol: 2 mg, Fiber: 3 g

Hummus and Date Bagel

Preparation time: 3 minutes/**Cooking Time:** 5 minutes /**Total time:** 10 minutes
Servings: 1/**Difficulty Level:** Medium
Ingredients:

- ¼ serving of Homemade Hummus/store-bought hummus
- 6 dates, pitted &halved
- 1 bagel
- Dash of salt & pepper

- ¼ cup of diced tomatoes
- 1 tbsp. of chives
- A squeeze of lemon juice
- 1 handful sprouts

Instructions:
The bagel is split in half. In a toaster or under the broiler, toast the bagel. Each side is rubbed with hummus. Add the salt, dates, and pepper to taste.

Nutritional Information:
Calories: 410 kcal, protein: 91 g, carbohydrates: 59 g, Fat: 2 g, Cholesterol: 0 mg, Fiber: 9.7 g

Curry Tofu Scramble

Preparation time: 5 minutes/**Cooking Time:** 5 minutes /**Total time:** 15 minutes
Servings: 3/**Difficulty Level:** Medium
Ingredients:
- 1 teaspoon of curry powder
- 1 teaspoon of olive oil
- 12oz. crumbled tofu,
- ¼ cup of skim milk
- ¼ teaspoon of chili flakes

Instructions
In a skillet, heat the olive oil. Toss in the tofu crumbles and chili flakes. Combine skim milk and curry powder in a mixing dish. Stir thoroughly after pouring the liquid over crumbled tofu. On medium-high heat, scramble the tofu for 3 minutes.

Nutritional Information:
Calories: 102 kcal, protein: 10 g, carbohydrates: 3.3 g, Fat: 6.4 g, Cholesterol: 0 mg, Fiber: 3 g

Breakfast Splits

Preparation time: 10 minutes/**Cooking Time:** 0 minutes/**Total time:** 10 minutes
Servings: 2/**Difficulty Level:** Easy
Ingredients:
- 2 tablespoons of low-fat yogurt

- 2 peeled bananas
- 4 tablespoons of granola
- 1 chopped strawberry
- ½ teaspoon of ground cinnamon

Instructions:
Combine yogurt, ground cinnamon, and strawberries in a mixing dish. Then cut the bananas lengthwise and fill them with the yogurt mass. Granola may be sprinkled on top of the fruits.

Nutritional Information:
Calories: 154 kcal, protein: 6.8 g, carbohydrates: 45.2 g, Fat: 8 g, Cholesterol: 1 mg, Fiber: 4 g

Tomato basil bruschetta

Preparation time: 5 minutes/**Cooking Time:** /**Total time:** 5 minutes
Servings: 6/**Difficulty Level:** Easy
Ingredients:
- 2 tablespoons of chopped basil
- 1/2 whole-grain baguette, six 1/2-inch-thick diagonal slices
- 1 tablespoon of chopped parsley
- 3 diced tomatoes,
- 2 minced cloves garlic,
- 1 teaspoon of olive oil
- 1/2 cup of diced fennel
- 1 teaspoon of black pepper
- 2 teaspoons of balsamic vinegar

Instructions:
Preheat the oven to 400 degrees Fahrenheit. Baguette pieces should be gently toasted. Combine all the remaining ingredients in a large mixing bowl. Distribute the mixture equally over the toasted bread. Serve right away.

Nutritional Information:
Calories: 142 kcal, protein: 5 g, carbohydrates: 26 g, Fat: 2 g, Cholesterol: 0 mg, Fiber: 2 g

Chapter 7: Smoothies and Drinks

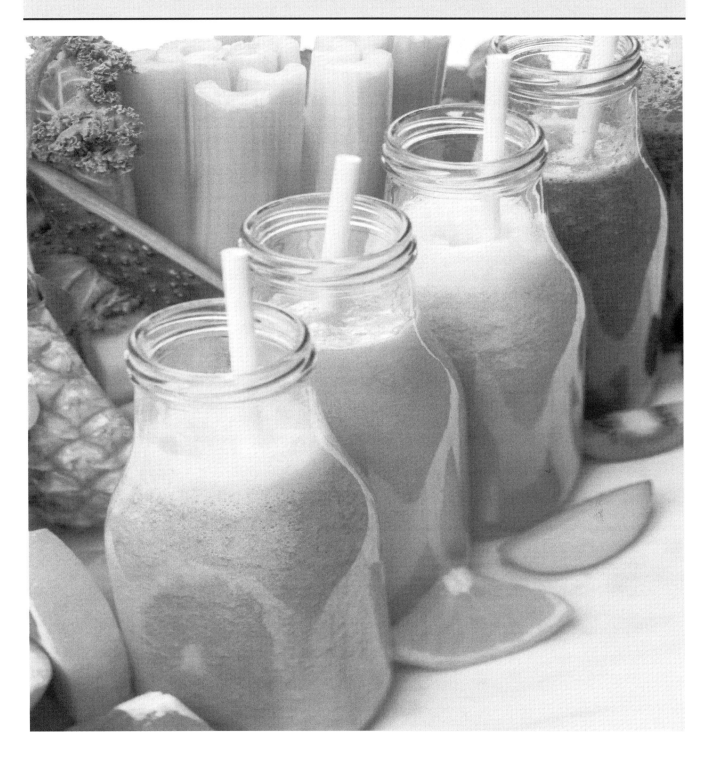

Mango Oat Smoothie

Preparation time: 5 minutes/**Cooking Time:** 0 minutes/**Total time:** 5 minutes

Servings: 3/**Difficulty Level:** Easy

Ingredients:
- 1/4 cup of old-fashioned oats
- 2 cups of frozen mango
- 1 banana: (frozen is better)
- 2 cups of oat milk /other plant-based milk /skim milk
- 1/4 lemon/orange (juiced)
- 1 tablespoon of ground flax seed

Instructions:
In a blender, combine all of the ingredients. Blend until completely smooth. Pour into three glasses and enjoy!

Nutritional Information:
Calories: 201 kcal, protein: 8 g, carbohydrates: 39 g, Fat: 3 g, Cholesterol: 3 mg, Fiber: 4 g

Avocado Island Green Smoothie

Preparation time: 5 minutes/**Cooking Time:** 0 minutes/**Total time:** 5 minutes

Servings: 1/**Difficulty Level:** Easy

Ingredients:
- ¼ medium avocado
- ½ cup of coconut milk
- 5.3-ounce coconut yogurt
- ½ cup of frozen pineapple
- 1 cup of power greens (any leafy greens)
- 1 tbsp. of ground flaxseed

Garnishes
- Optional: 1 wedge of fresh pineapple

- ½ tbsp. of shredded coconut optional

Instructions:
Simply combine the ingredients in a blender and mix until smooth.

Nutritional Information:
Calories: 339 kcal, protein: 19 g, carbohydrates: 34 g, Fat: 16 g, Cholesterol: 10 mg, Fiber: 8 g

Pumpkin Pie Smoothie

Preparation time: 5 minutes/**Cooking Time:** 0 minutes/**Total time:** 5 minutes

Servings: 1/**Difficulty Level:** Easy

Ingredients:
- 1 medium frozen banana
- 1 cup of light vanilla almond milk or milk of choice
- 1/4 cup of ice
- 1/2 tsp of pumpkin pie spice*
- 1 scoop of vanilla protein powder
- 1/8 tsp of cinnamon
- 1 tbsp. of almond butter
- 1/4 cup of canned pumpkin puree

*If you don't have pumpkin pie spice, make your own by combining 1/4 teaspoon of ground nutmeg, ground cloves, & ground allspice.

Instructions:
Simply combine the ingredients in a blender and mix until smooth.

Nutritional Information:
Calories: 393 kcal, protein: 30 g, carbohydrates: 49 g, Fat: 12 g, Cholesterol: 40 mg, Fiber: 6 g

Vegan Tropical Smoothie

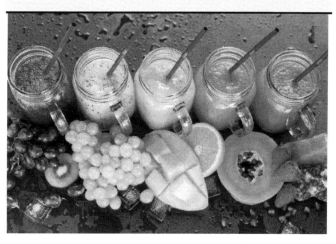

Preparation time: 5 minutes/**Cooking Time:** 0 minutes /**Total time:** 5 minutes

Servings: 2/**Difficulty Level:** Easy

Ingredients:
- 1 large frozen banana

- ¼ cup of Silken tofu
- 1 cup of almond milk
- 1 ½ cup of frozen strawberry
- 1½ cup of frozen mango¼ cup of water (more or less may require depending on preference)
- 2 Tbsp. of hemp seeds

Instructions:
Toss all ingredients into a blender, except the water, and mix until desired consistency is reached.

Nutritional Information:
Calories: 279 kcal, protein: 3 g, carbohydrates: 39 g, Fat: 15 g, Cholesterol: 9 mg, Fiber: 5 g

Strawberry Rhubarb Pie Smoothie

Preparation time: 5 minutes/**Cooking Time:** 0 minutes/**Total time:** 5 minutes

Servings: 1/**Difficulty Level:** Easy

Ingredients:
- 1/2 cup of chopped rhubarb
- 1 cup of frozen sliced strawberries
- 1 small or 1/2 medium banana; (1/2 cup of sliced), ideally frozen
- 3 tablespoons of rolled oats
- 1 tablespoon of slivered almonds
- 1 tablespoon of maple syrup
- Optional: nutty granola; for topping
- 1 cup of unsweetened coconut milk beverage
- Ice, as needed
- 1 teaspoon of vanilla

Instructions:
Combine all ingredients in a blender and blend until smooth. As required, add ice to the mix. Top with your favorite nutty granola, if desired.

Nutritional Information:
Calories: 372 kcal, protein: 8 g, carbohydrates: 31 g, Fat: 27 g, Cholesterol: 10 mg, Fiber: 4 g

Berry Coconut Water Smoothie

Preparation time: 5 minutes/**Cooking Time:** 0 minutes/**Total time:** 5 minutes

Servings: 2/**Difficulty Level:** Easy

Ingredients:
- 2 tablespoons of warm water
- ¼ cup of goji berries
- 3 cups of frozen berries
- 1 teaspoon of ground cinnamon
- 1 cup of Unsweetened Coconut milk/ Yogurt Alternative
- 1 banana
- 1 cup of coconut water

Optional for serving:
- Fresh berries
- Granola; (homemade/store-bought)

Instructions:
In a blender container, combine the goji berries and water and mix for 30 seconds, or until smooth. If necessary, scrape down the sides of the blender with a spatula. Blend on high for 2 minutes, or until smooth and creamy, adding coconut milk/yogurt alternatives, coconut water, banana, frozen berries, and cinnamon to the blender container. Transfer to glasses and, if preferred, top with granola and fresh berries.

Nutritional Information:
Calories: 390 kcal, protein: 5.3 g, carbohydrates: 59.6 g, Fat: 5.3 g, Cholesterol: 10 mg, Fiber: 14.2 g

Orange Mango Sunshine Smoothie

Preparation time: 5 minutes/**Cooking Time:** 5 minutes/**Total time:** 10 minutes

Servings: 2/**Difficulty Level:** Easy

Ingredients:
- 1 Mango (2 cups; cubes)
- 2 Oranges; segments only
- 1 medium Carrot
- 1/2-1 tsp of minced, fresh Ginger
- 1 cup of Unsweetened Soy Milk/milk of choice
- 1 cup of Ice
- 1/4 tsp of Turmeric

Instructions:
Blend all the ingredients in a high-powered blender until smooth. If preferred, top with a sprinkling of cinnamon.

Nutritional Information:
Calories: 248 kcal, protein: 6.7 g, carbohydrates: 54.4 g, Fat: 2.9 g, Cholesterol: 0 mg, Fiber: 7.8 g

Banana Nut Smoothie

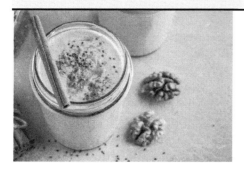

Preparation time: 5 minutes/**Cooking Time:** /**Total time:** 5 minutes

Servings: 1/**Difficulty Level:** Easy

Ingredients:
- 2 Tbsp. of Almond Butter
- 1 Banana frozen
- 1/2 tsp of Cinnamon
- 1 cup of Almond Milk unsweetened
- 1 tsp of Maple Syrup
- 1 Tbsp. of Flaxseed ground; (optional)

Instructions:
Combine all ingredients in a blender and blend until smooth. If desired, sprinkle with cinnamon. Serve right away.

Nutritional Information:
Calories: 412 kcal, protein: 11 g, carbohydrates: 43 g, Fat: 25 g, Cholesterol: 2.5 mg, Fiber: 11 g

Carrot Banana Smoothie

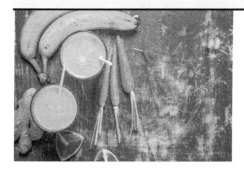

Preparation time: 5 minutes/**Cooking Time:** 0 minutes/**Total time:** 5 minutes

Servings: 1/**Difficulty Level:** Easy

Ingredients:
- ¼ cup of oats

- 1 cup of dairy-free milk: protein added milk /soy milk
- ☐ cup of shredded carrots
- 1 tablespoon of walnuts
- 1 tablespoon of raisins
- ½ frozen banana; about ½ cup of frozen slices
- 1 tablespoon of ground flaxseed
- 1 scoop of vanilla protein powder
- 1 teaspoon of ground cinnamon

Instructions:
Combine all ingredients except the protein powder and frozen bananas in a blender. Stir or shake the mixture and set aside for 10 minutes. Combine the protein powder with the frozen bananas. Blend until the mixture is smooth and creamy.

Nutritional Information:
Calories: 379 kcal, protein: 25 g, carbohydrates: 40 g, Fat: 16 g, Cholesterol: 0 mg, Fiber: 11 g

Healthy Blueberry Smoothie with Almond Butter

Preparation time: 3 minutes/**Cooking Time:** 0 minutes/**Total time:** 3 minutes

Servings: 1/**Difficulty Level:** Easy

Ingredients:
- 1/2 banana
- 1/2 cup of blueberries
- 1 tbsp. of almond butter
- 6 oz. vanilla soy milk
- 1 tbsp. of cocoa powder
- ¼ teaspoon of cinnamon
- ½ cup of ice chips
- 1 tbsp. of flaxseed ground

Instructions:
In a blender cup, combine all of the ingredients. Blend for 10 seconds or until the mixture is completely smooth.

Nutritional Information:
Calories: 338 kcal, protein: 11.7 g, carbohydrates: 42.9 g, Fat: 16.7 g, Cholesterol: 0 mg, Fiber: 10.8 g

Morning Glory Smoothie

Preparation time: 5 minutes/**Cooking Time:** 0 minutes /**Total time:** 5 minutes
Servings: 2/**Difficulty Level:** Easy

Ingredients:
- 1 cup of milk
- ½ cup of apple juice
- 2 tablespoons of walnuts
- 2 tablespoons of unsweetened coconut flakes
- 2 frozen bananas
- 1 small carrot
- ½ teaspoon ground cinnamon
- ½ teaspoon of pure vanilla extract
- ½ teaspoon of stevia
- 1-2 cups of ice cubes

Instructions:
Combine the milk, walnuts, apple juice, and coconut flakes in a blender mixer. Allow for 5 minutes of resting time. Add the frozen bananas, cinnamon, carrots, stevia, vanilla essence, and ice cubes in a pitcher. Puree until completely smooth. Serve right away.

Nutritional Information:
Calories: 276 kcal, protein: 6 g, carbohydrates: 46 g, Fat: 8 g, Cholesterol: 2 mg, Fiber: 6 g

Celery Smoothie with Apple and Banana

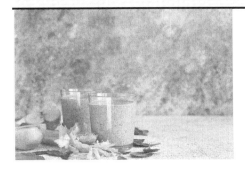

Preparation time: 5 minutes/**Cooking Time:** 0 minutes /**Total time:** 5 minutes

Servings: 2/**Difficulty Level:** Easy

Ingredients:
- 1 cup of baby spinach
- 1 cup of chopped celery: preferably frozen
- 1 green apple: cored & cut into chunks
- 1 frozen banana
- ½ avocado
- 1 tablespoon lemon juice
- Dash of vanilla extract
- 1 teaspoon of freshly grated ginger

Instructions:
Combine all ingredients in a blender. Add about ¾ to 1 cup water. Blend until smooth, and enjoy!

Nutritional Information:
Calories: 194 kcal, protein: 3 g, carbohydrates: 33 g, Fat: 8 g, Cholesterol: 1 mg, Fiber: 8 g

Green Smoothie with Chia and Peach

Preparation time: 5 minutes/**Cooking Time:** 0 minutes /**Total time:** 5 minutes

Servings: 2/**Difficulty Level:** Easy

Ingredients:
- 1 tbsp. of chia seeds
- 1 banana ripe, ideally frozen
- 1 peach chopped, ripe
- 1 cup of unsweetened almond milk cold
- 1 cup of spinach fresh, washed

Instructions:
In a blender, combine the ingredients in the order stated (you want your greens on the bottom by the blade, so they blend better and have the chia on the bottom to absorb some liquid before you blend). Allow for a few minutes for the chia seeds to absorb the almond milk. Combine all ingredients in a blender and serve with your preferred toppings. Enjoy!

Nutritional Information:
Calories: 241 kcal, protein: 6 g, carbohydrates: 43 g, Fat: 7 g, Cholesterol: 1 mg, Fiber: 10 g

Green Grapefruit Smoothie

Preparation time: 5 minutes/**Cooking Time:** 0 minutes /**Total time:** 5 minutes

Servings: 1/**Difficulty Level:** Easy

Ingredients:
- ½ grapefruit - wedges and juice, see directions

- 2 kale leaves - stems removed and roughly torn, about 2 cups loosely packed
- 1 banana - peeled and frozen
- 1 tablespoon of chia seeds
- ½ cup water - more if needed

Instructions:
To prepare the grapefruit, slice in half and cut out the wedges of one half. Transfer the wedges and whatever leftover juice you can squeeze out of the grapefruit half you used to the blender.

Add the kale leaves, banana, chia seeds, and water. Blend at high speed for about 30 seconds to 1 minute or until smooth. Add more water if needed. If you do not use a frozen banana, consider adding ice to make it colder. Enjoy!

Nutritional Information:
Calories: 281 kcal, protein: 10 g, carbohydrates: 57 g, Fat: 6 g, Cholesterol: 0 mg, Fiber: 9 g

Green Smoothie with Matcha Chia Smoothie

Preparation time: 5 minutes/**Cooking Time:** 0 minutes /**Total time:** 5 minutes

Servings: 1/**Difficulty Level:** Easy

Ingredients:
- 1/4 cup of baby spinach
- 2 tablespoons of unsweetened coconut water
- 1/2 large frozen banana
- 1 teaspoon of match a green tea powder
- 1/2 teaspoon of pure vanilla extract
- 1 teaspoon of chia seeds
- 1 cup of unsweetened milk of choice (soy, almond, or oat)

Instructions:
Blend the spinach with coconut water until the spinach is completely pureed. Blend in the remaining ingredients until smooth. If desired, add more milk and ice.

Nutritional Information:
Calories: 168 kcal, protein: 8 g, carbohydrates: 31 g, Fat: 4 g, Cholesterol: 2 mg, Fiber: 7 g

Blueberry Pineapple Smoothie

Preparation time: 5 minutes/**Cooking Time:** 0 minutes /**Total time:** 5 minutes

Servings: 2/**Difficulty Level:** Easy

Ingredients:
- 1 cup of blueberries (fresh or frozen)
- 1 cup of pineapple chunks (fresh or frozen)
- 2 cups of frozen banana slices
- 1/2 cup of unsweetened vanilla almond milk, divided
- 1/2 cup of vanilla Greek yogurt

Instructions:
Combine almond milk, blueberries, banana, pineapple, and Greek yogurt to make the blueberry pineapple smoothie in a blender. Cover and mix until completely smooth, scraping down the edges as needed. In large glasses, divide blueberry pineapple smoothie and top with more blueberries and pineapple chunks. Enjoy!

Nutritional Information:
Calories: 236.7 kcal, protein: 5.68 g, carbohydrates: 52.06 g, Fat: 2.75 g, Cholesterol: 6.3 mg, Fiber: 5.22 g

Beet Smoothie

Preparation time: 4 minutes/**Cooking Time:** 1 minute /**Total time:** 5 minutes

Servings: 2/**Difficulty Level:** Easy

Ingredients:
- 1/2 cup of unsweetened almond milk or milk of choice
- 1 cup of mixed frozen blueberries/mixed berries
- 1 small beet peeled & diced: (about 8 ounces)
- Optional sweetener: 1-2 teaspoons honey plus additional to taste (use agave to make vegan)
- 1/4 cup of frozen pineapple
- 1/4 cup off plain nonfat Greek yogurt use non-dairy yogurt to make vegan
- Optional mix-ins: chia seeds, hempseed, and ground flaxseed (I like mine with a sprinkle of chia or hempseed; hempseed is what you see pictured in the photos); I also like to add 2 tablespoons oatmeal to make the smoothie even more filling.

Instructions:
Combine the beet, blueberries, pineapple, almond milk, and Greek yogurt in a high-powered blender. Blend until completely smooth. Add honey or date and mix it again if you want a sweeter smoothie. Enjoy right away or keep refrigerated for up to one day.

Nutritional Information:
Calories: 95 kcal, protein: 4 g, carbohydrates: 19 g, Fat: 1 g, Cholesterol: 2 mg, Fiber: 4 g

Chocolate Strawberry Banana Smoothie

Preparation time: 5 minutes/**Cooking Time:** 0 minutes /**Total time:** 5 minutes

Servings: 2/**Difficulty Level:** Easy

Ingredients:
- ½ cup of Yogurt
- 1 Frozen Banana (approx. ½ cup)
- ½ cup of Strawberries
- 2 tbsp. of Unsweetened Cocoa Powder
- ½ tsp of Vanilla Essence
- 1 tbsp. of honey (or as needed)
- ½ cup of Milk

Instructions:
Combine the yogurt, frozen banana, chopped strawberries, cocoa powder, vanilla, honey, and milk in a blender. Blend everything until smooth. Pour into glasses and serve.

Nutritional Information:
Calories: 185 kcal, protein: 6 g, carbohydrates: 33 g, Fat: 5 g, Cholesterol: 14 mg, Fiber: 4 g

Ginger Spice Smoothie

Preparation time: 5 minutes/**Cooking Time:** 0 minutes /**Total time:** 5 minutes

Servings: 1/**Difficulty Level:** Easy

Ingredients:
- 1/2 cups of almond/cashew milk
- 2 tablespoons of raw almond butter
- 1/4 teaspoon of grated nutmeg
- 1 handful baby spinach/greens of choice
- 2 teaspoons of grated ginger

Instructions:
Place all ingredients in a blender and blend until smooth and creamy. Serve immediately.

Nutritional Information:
Calories: 400 kcal, protein: 13 g, carbohydrates: 19 g, Fat: 31 g, Cholesterol: 0 mg, Fiber: 7 g

Avocado Blueberry Smoothie

Preparation time: 5 minutes/**Cooking Time:** 0 minutes /**Total time:** 5 minutes

Servings: 2/**Difficulty Level:** Easy

Ingredients:
- 1 1/2 cups of blueberries frozen
- 3/4 cup of almond milk unsweetened
- 1 cup of baby spinach
- 1/2 cup of ice
- 1/2 avocado peeled
- 1/2 cup of yogurt unsweetened, or Greek (full fat preferred)
- 10-gram whey protein
- 2 tablespoons of coconut unsweetened

Instructions:
Add all ingredients to a blender and process until thick and creamy. Taste, and use 1-2 tablespoons of your favorite sweetener, if necessary.

Nutritional Information:
Calories: 215 kcal, protein: 5 g, carbohydrates: 25 g, Fat: 13 g, Cholesterol: 8 mg, Fiber: 7 g

Oatmeal Smoothie

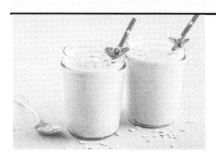

Preparation time: 5 minutes/**Cooking Time:** 0 minutes /**Total time:** 5 minutes

Servings: 1/**Difficulty Level:** Easy

Ingredients:

- 1/4 cup of rolled_oats
- 1 frozen banana (sliced)
- 2 tablespoons of peanut butter
- 1 tablespoon of ground_flax_seeds
- 3/4 cup of almond milk or water
- ½ to 1 tablespoon of maple_syrup (or to taste)
- 3 to 5 ice cubes

Instructions:

In a high-speed blender, add the oats and blend briefly to break them down into smaller pieces. This will prevent you from finding any big chunks of oatmeal in your smoothie later. If desired, add in the banana, peanut butter, flax, liquid, and maple syrup, then blend until smooth. Add the ice cubes and blend again until the smoothie has a slushy texture. Serve right away for the best taste and texture.

Nutritional Information:
Calories: 461 kcal, protein: 14 g, carbohydrates: 56 g, Fat: 23 g, Cholesterol: 2 mg, Fiber: 10 g

Cranberry Orange Smoothie

Preparation time: 5 minutes/**Cooking Time:** 0 minutes /**Total time:** 5 minutes

Servings: 2/**Difficulty Level:** Easy

Ingredients:
- 1/2 cup of cranberry sauce
- 1/2 cup of orange juice
- 1 cup of plain nonfat yogurt
- 1 cup of banana, sliced
- 1/2 cup of skim milk

Instructions:
Combine all ingredients in a blender and process until smooth.

Nutritional Information:
Calories: 326 kcal, protein: 11 g, carbohydrates: 72 g, Fat: 1 g, Cholesterol: 4 mg, Fiber: 4 g

Banana Melon Smoothies

Preparation time: 5 minutes/**Cooking Time:** 0 minutes /**Total time:** 5 minutes

Servings: 2/**Difficulty Level:** Easy

Ingredients:

- 6 ounces soft tofu
- 1 banana
- 1 cup of cantaloupe
- 1/2 cup of skim milk
- 1/2 cup of apple juice

Instructions:
Place all ingredients in a blender and process until smooth.

Nutritional Information:
Calories: 230 kcal, protein: 9 g, carbohydrates: 46 g, Fat: 3 g, Cholesterol: 1 mg, Fiber: 4 g

Peach Smoothies

Preparation time: 5 minutes/**Cooking Time:** 0 minutes /**Total time:** 5 minutes

Servings: 1/**Difficulty Level:** Easy

Ingredients:
- 1 cup of banana, sliced
- 1 cup of orange juice
- 1 cup low-fat vanilla yogurt
- 3/4 cup of peaches, sliced and frozen

Instructions:
Place all ingredients in a blender and process until thick and smooth.

Nutritional Information:
Calories: 563 kcal, protein: 18 g, carbohydrates: 121 g, Fat: 5 g, Cholesterol: 12 mg, Fiber: 8 g

Honeydew Smoothie Bowl

Preparation time: 5 minutes/**Cooking Time:** 0 minutes /**Total time:** 5 minutes

Servings: 2/**Difficulty Level:** Easy

Ingredients:
- 4 cups of frozen cubed honeydew: 1/2-inch pieces
- ½ cup of unsweetened coconut milk beverage
- □ cup of green juice, such as wheatgrass
- Pinch of salt
- 1 tablespoon of honey
- Melon balls, nuts berries, and fresh basil for garnish

Instructions:

Combine honeydew, coconut milk, juice, honey, and salt in a food processor or high-speed blender. Alternate between pulsing and blending, stopping to stir and scrape down the sides as needed, until thick and smooth, 1 to 2 minutes. If desired, serve the smoothie topped with more melon, berries, nuts, and basil.

Nutritional Information:
Calories: 176 kcal, protein: 2.5 g, carbohydrates: 41.1 g, Fat: 1.6 g, Cholesterol: 18 mg, Fiber: 3 g

Peanut Butter & Jelly Smoothie

Preparation time: 5 minutes/**Cooking Time:** 0 minutes /**Total time:** 5 minutes

Servings: 1/**Difficulty Level:** Easy

Ingredients:
- ½ cup of low-fat milk
- □ cup of no-fat plain Greek yogurt
- 1 cup of baby spinach
- 1 cup of frozen banana slices (about 1 medium banana)
- ½ cup of frozen strawberries
- 1 tablespoon of natural peanut butter
- 1-2 teaspoons of pure maple syrup or honey (optional)

Instructions:
In a blender, combine the yogurt and milk, add the spinach, strawberries, peanut butter, banana, and sweetener (if using), mix until smooth.

Nutritional Information:
Calories: 367 kcal, protein: 18.1 g, carbohydrates: 53.9 g, Fat: 10.2 g, Cholesterol: 9.9 mg, Fiber: 7.1 g

Orange Flax Smoothie

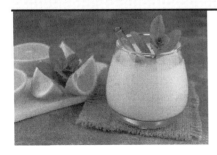

Preparation time: 5 minutes/**Cooking Time:** 0 minutes /**Total time:** 5 minutes

Servings: 2/**Difficulty Level:** Easy

Ingredients:
- 2 tablespoons of ground flaxseed
- 2 cups of frozen peach slices
- 1 cup of orange juice
- 1 tablespoon of chopped fresh ginger
- 1 cup of carrot juice

Instructions:
Combine peaches, carrot juice, orange juice, flaxseed, and ginger in a blender, blend until smooth. Serve immediately.

Nutritional Information:
Calories: 209 kcal, protein: 4.9 g, carbohydrates: 41.4 g, Fat: 4.3 g, Cholesterol: 2 mg, Fiber: 5.7 g

Mermaid Smoothie Bowl

Preparation time: 5 minutes/**Cooking Time:** 0 minutes /**Total time:** 5 minutes

Servings: 2/**Difficulty Level:** Easy

Ingredients:
- 2 frozen bananas, peeled
- 2 kiwis, peeled
- 1 cup of fresh pineapple chunks
- ½ cup of fresh blueberries
- 1 cup of almond milk
- 2 teaspoons of blue spirulina powder
- ½ small Fuji apple, thinly sliced and cut into 1-inch flower shapes

Instructions:
Combine kiwis, bananas, almond milk, pineapple, and spirulina in a blender. Blend on high for 2 minutes, or until smooth. Pour the smoothie into two bowls. Add blueberries and apples on the top.

Nutritional Information:
Calories: 251 kcal, protein: 4.8 g, carbohydrates: 59.5 g, Fat: 2.5 g, Cholesterol: 2 mg, Fiber: 8.7 g

Guava Smoothie

Preparation time: 5 minutes/**Cooking Time:** 0 minutes /**Total time:** 5 minutes

Servings: 2/**Difficulty Level:** Easy

Ingredients:
- 1 cup of baby spinach finely chopped.
- 1 banana peeled and sliced.

- 1 cup of guava, seeds removed, chopped.
- 1 tsp of fresh ginger, grated.
- 2 cups of water
- ½ medium-sized mango, peeled and chopped.

Instructions:

Peel the guava and cut it in half. Scoop out the seeds and wash them. Cut into small pieces and set aside. Rinse the baby spinach thoroughly under cold running water. Drain well and torn into small pieces. Set aside. Peel the banana and chop it into small chunks. Set aside. Peel the mango and cut it into small pieces. Set aside. Now, combine guava, baby spinach, banana, ginger, and mango in a juicer and process until well combined. Gradually add water and blend until all combine and creamy. Transfer to a serving glass and refrigerate for 20 minutes before serving. Enjoy!

Nutritional Information:

Calories: 166 kcal, protein: 3.9 g, carbohydrates: 39.1 g, Fat: 1.4 g, Cholesterol: 0 mg, Fiber: 7.8 g

Pear and Arugula Smoothie

Preparation time: 5 minutes/**Cooking Time:** 0 minutes /**Total time:** 5 minutes

Servings: 1/**Difficulty Level:** Easy

Ingredients:
- 1 tablespoon of almonds, pine nuts, or walnuts
- 1/2 ripe cored pear,

- 1/4 cup of Greek yogurt (fat-free)
- 1/2 cup of freshly squeezed orange juice
- 1 1/4- inch peeled slice of fresh ginger,
- 3 – 4 ice cubes
- 1 cup of tightly packed arugula,

Instructions:

In a blender, combine all ingredients and mix until smooth (for about 1 minute). Serve it.

Nutritional Information:

Calories: 207 kcal, protein: 5 g, carbohydrates: 36 g, Fat: 5 g, Cholesterol: 2 mg, Fiber:4 g

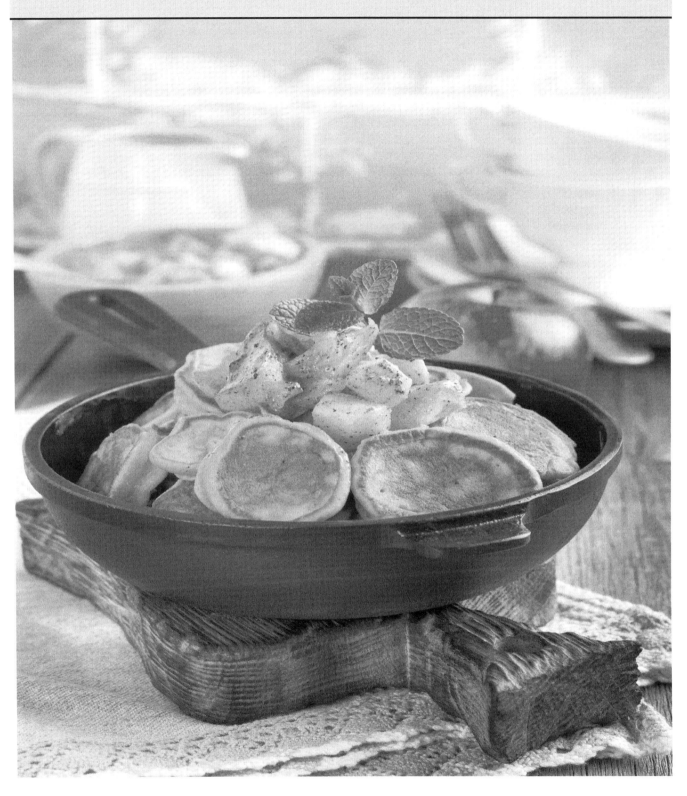

Old Bay Crispy Kale Chips

Preparation time: 10 minutes/**Cooking Time:** 25 minutes/**Total time:** 35minutes
Servings: 4/**Difficulty Level:** Easy
Ingredients:
- bunch kale, washed
- tablespoons olive oil
- 1 to 3 teaspoons Old Bay Seasoning
- Sea salt, to taste

Instructions:
Preheat the oven to 300 ℉. Remove the kale's tough stems and shred the leaves into large pieces. Combine all of the ingredients in a large mixing bowl. Toss with olive oil and spices to coat. Arrange the leaves on prepared baking sheets in a single layer.
Bake for 10 minutes, uncovered, before rotating pans. Bake for a further 15 minutes, or until crisp and beginning to brown. Allow at least 5 minutes to stand before serving.
Nutritional Information:
Calories: 101 kcal, protein: 3 g, carbohydrates: 8 g, Fat: 7 g, Cholesterol: 0 mg, Fiber: 2 g

Nutty Broccoli Slaw

Preparation time: 15 minutes/**Cooking Time:** 0 minutes/**Total time:** 15 minutes
Servings: 16/**Difficulty Level:** Easy
Ingredients:
- 2 cups of sliced green onions: 2 bunches
- package of chicken ramen noodles; (3 ounces)
- 1-1/2 cups of broccoli florets
- 1 package of broccoli coleslaw mix; (16 ounces)
- 1 can of ripe olives (6 ounces); drained and halved
- 1 cup of sunflower kernels, toasted
- 1/2 cup of slivered almonds, toasted
- 1/2 cup cider vinegar
- 1/2 cup of sugar
- 1/2 cup olive oil

Instructions:
Open the noodle seasoning package and put the crushed noodles in a large mixing bowl. Combine the onions, sunflower kernels, broccoli, slaw mix, olives, and almonds. Combine the seasoning package's oil, vinegar, sugar, and contents in a jar with a tight-fitting cover; shake thoroughly. Drizzle the dressing over salad and toss to combine. Serve right away.
Nutritional Information:

Calories: 206 kcal, protein: 4 g, carbohydrates: 16 g, Fat: 15 g, Cholesterol: 0 mg, Fiber: 3 g

Chipotle Lime Avocado Salad

Preparation time: 15 minutes/**Cooking Time:** 0 minutes/**Total time:** 15 minutes
Servings: 4/**Difficulty Level:** Easy
Ingredients:
- 1/4 cup lime juice
- 1/4 cup of maple syrup
- 1/2 teaspoon chipotle pepper, ground
- 1/4 teaspoon cayenne pepper
- 2 peeled and sliced medium ripe avocados
- peeled and sliced 1/2 a medium cucumber
- a tablespoon fresh chives, minced
- large tomatoes, peeled and cut into 1/2-inch thick slices

Instructions:
Whisk lime juice, maple syrup, chipotle pepper, and, if preferred, cayenne pepper together in a small bowl until well combined. Combine avocados, cucumber, and chives in a separate bowl. Drizzle dressing over the salad and gently mix to coat. Serve with tomatoes on the side.
Nutritional Information:
Calories: 191 kcal, protein: 3 g, carbohydrates: 25 g, Fat: 11 g, Cholesterol: 0 mg, Fiber: 6 g

Nuts and Seeds Trail Mix

Preparation time: 5 minutes/**Cooking Time:** 0 minutes/**Total time:** 5 minutes
Servings: 5 cups/**Difficulty Level:** Easy
Ingredients:
- cup salted pumpkin seeds or petites
- 1 cup unbranched almonds
- 1 cup unsalted sunflower kernels
- 1 cup walnut halves
- 1 cup dried apricots
- 1 cup dark chocolate chips

Instructions:
Place all ingredients in a large bowl; toss to combine. Store in an airtight container.
Nutritional Information:
Calories: 336 kcal, protein: 11 g, carbohydrates: 22 g, Fat: 25 g, Cholesterol: 0 mg, Fiber: 4 g

Hummus

Preparation time: 25 minutes/**Cooking Time:** 20 minutes plus chilling
Total time: 1 hour 15 minutes/**Servings:** 1 1/2 cup/**Difficulty Level:** Easy
Ingredients:

- 1/4 cup of fresh lemon juice
- 1/2 teaspoon of baking soda
- 1/2 teaspoon of kosher salt
- can (15 ounces) garbanzo beans/chickpeas: rinsed & drained
- 1 tablespoon of minced garlic
- 1/2 cup of tahini
- 1/2 teaspoon of ground cumin
- tablespoons of extra virgin olive oil
- Optional: roasted garbanzo beans, Olive oil, ground sumac, toasted sesame seeds,
- 1/4 cup of cold water

Instructions:
Place the garbanzo beans and enough water to cover them by 1 inch in a large saucepan. Rub the beans together gently to release the outer skin. Pour off the water as well as any floating skins. Drain after repeating steps 2-3 times unless no skins float to the top. Return to saucepan; stir in baking soda and 1 inch of water. Bring to a boil, then turn off the heat. Cook, uncovered, for 20-25 minutes, or until beans are soft and begin to come apart.
Meanwhile, puree the garlic, lemon juice, and salt in a blender until smooth. Allow 10 minutes to stand before straining and discarding the solids. Cumin is added at this point. Combine tahini and olive oil in a small bowl.
Blend the beans with the cold water in a blender. Cover loosely with cover and process until absolutely smooth. Stir in the lemon mixture in the food processor. Slowly drizzle in the tahini mixture while the blender runs, scraping down the sides as required. If desired, add more salt and cumin to the seasoning. Refrigerate for at least 30 minutes after transferring the mixture to the serving bowl. Additional toppings or olive oil may be added if desired.

Nutritional Information:
Calories: 250 kcal, protein: 7 g, carbohydrates: 15 g, Fat: 19 g, Cholesterol: 0 mg, Fiber: 5 g

Honey-Lime Berry Salad

Preparation time: 15 minutes/**Cooking Time:** 0 minutes/**Total time:** 15 minutes
Servings: 10/**Difficulty Level:** Easy
Ingredients:

- 4 cups fresh strawberries, halved
- cups fresh blueberries
- medium Granny Smith apples, cubed
- 1/3 cup lime juice
- 1/4 to 1/3 cup honey
- 2 tablespoons minced fresh mint

Instructions:
Combine strawberries, blueberries, and apples in a large mixing dish. Combine the lime juice, honey, and mint in a small mixing bowl. Toss the fruit in the dressing to coat.

Nutritional Information:
Calories: 93 kcal, protein: 1 g, carbohydrates: 24 g, Fat: 0 g, Cholesterol: 0 mg, Fiber: 3 g

Smoky Cauliflower

Preparation time: 30 minutes/**Cooking Time:** 0 minutes/**Total time:** 30 minutes
Servings: 8/**Difficulty Level:** Easy
Ingredients:

- tablespoons of olive oil
- 1 large head cauliflower: 1-inch florets: about 9 cups
- 3/4 teaspoon of salt
- 1 teaspoon of smoked paprika
- tablespoons of minced fresh parsley
- 2 garlic cloves: minced

Instructions:
In a large mixing bowl, place the cauliflower. Combine the oil, paprika, and salt. Drizzle the dressing over the cauliflower and toss to coat. Fill a 15x10x1-inch baking pan halfway with the batter. Bake for 10 minutes at 450°F, uncovered. Add the garlic and mix well. Bake for another 10-15 minutes, stirring periodically, or until cauliflower is soft and lightly browned. Serve with a parsley garnish.

Nutritional Information:
Calories: 58 kcal, protein: 2 g, carbohydrates: 6 g, Fat: 4 g, Cholesterol: 0 mg, Fiber: 3 g

Chewy Granola Bars

Preparation time: 10 minutes/**Cooking Time:** 25 minutes plus cooling /**Total time:** 40 minutes/**Servings:** 2 dozen/**Difficulty Level:** Medium
Ingredients:

- 1/2 cup butter, softened

- 1 cup packed brown sugar
- 1/4 cup sugar
- 1 large egg, room temperature
- tablespoons honey
- 1/2 teaspoon vanilla extract
- 1 cup all-purpose flour
- 1 teaspoon ground cinnamon
- 1/2 teaspoon baking powder
- 1/4 teaspoon salt
- 1-1/2 cups quick-cooking oats
- 1-1/4 cups Rice Krispies
- 1 cup chopped nuts

- Optional: Raisins or semisweet chocolate chips (1 cup each)

Instructions:
Preheat oven to 350°F. Cream butter and sugars until light and fluffy, 5-7 minutes. Beat in egg, honey, and vanilla. Whisk together flour, cinnamon, baking powder, and salt; gradually beat into creamed mixture. Stir in oats, Rice Krispies, nuts, raisins, or chocolate chips. Press into a greased 13x9-in. pan. Bake until light brown, 25-30 minutes. Cool on a wire rack. Cut into bars.

Nutritional Information:
Calories: 160 kcal, protein: 3 g, carbohydrates: 22 g, Fat: 7 g, Cholesterol: 19 mg, Fiber: 1 g

Mango Black Bean Salsa

Preparation time: 15 minutes/**Cooking Time:** 0 minutes /**Total time:** 15 minutes
Servings: 12/**Difficulty Level:** Medium
Ingredients:
- 1 can (15 ounces) black beans, rinsed and drained
- 1 can (11 ounces) Mexico, drained
- 1 medium mango, peeled and cubed
- 1/4 cup finely chopped onion
- 1/4 cup minced fresh cilantro
- tablespoons lime juice
- 1 teaspoon garlic salt
- 1/4 teaspoon ground cumin
- Baked tortilla chip scoops

Instructions:
In a large bowl, mix all ingredients except chips. Refrigerate until serving. Serve with chips.
Nutritional Information:
Calories: 70 kcal, protein: 3 g, carbohydrates: 14 g, Fat: 0 g, Cholesterol: 0 mg, Fiber: 2 g

Homemade Guacamole

Preparation time: 10 minutes/**Cooking Time:** 0 minutes /**Total time:** 10 minutes
Servings: 2 cups/**Difficulty Level:** Medium
Ingredients:
- medium ripe avocados, peeled and cubed
- 1 garlic clove, minced
- 1/4 to 1/2 teaspoon salt
- 1 small onion, finely chopped
- 1 to 2 tablespoons lime juice
- 1 tablespoon minced fresh cilantro
- medium tomatoes, seeded and chopped, optional
- 1/4 cup mayonnaise, optional

Instructions:
Mash avocados with garlic and salt. Stir in remaining ingredients, adding tomatoes and mayonnaise if desired.
Nutritional Information:
Calories: 90 kcal, protein: 1 g, carbohydrates: 6 g, Fat: 8 g, Cholesterol: 0 mg, Fiber: 4 g

Apple Chips

Preparation time: 20 minutes/**Cooking Time:** 2 hours /**Total time:** 2 hours 40 minutes/**Servings:** 4/**Difficulty Level:** Medium
Ingredients:
- 1 teaspoon of ground cinnamon
- large apples, such as Honey crisp, Fuji, or Gala

Instructions:
Preheat the oven to 200 degrees Fahrenheit. Use a silicone baking mat or parchment paper to line two large baking sheets.
Using a mandolin, finely slice the apples to approximately 1/8-inch thick. Each slice should have the seeds removed. On the baking sheets, arrange the apple slices in a single layer. Cinnamon should be sprinkled on both sides, and bake the apples for one hour—Bake for another hour after flipping the apples. Please turn off the oven and allow the apples to cool for approximately 30 minutes before removing them. Continue baking the apples for 15 minutes if they are not crispy.
Take the apples off the baking pan, eat them right away, or keep them in the airtight container.
Nutritional Information:
Calories: 88 kcal, protein: 1 g, carbohydrates: 24 g, Fat: 1 g, Cholesterol: 0 mg, Fiber: 2.7 g

Pita Chips

Preparation time: 10 minutes/**Cooking Time:** 10 minutes /**Total time:** 20 minutes
Servings: 4/**Difficulty Level:** Easy
Ingredients:
- 1/4 tsp of garlic powder
- 1 Tbsp. of grated Parmesan cheese
- 1/2 tsp of salt
- Cooking spray
- 1 Tbsp. of dried Italian seasoning
- (6-inch) pita bread (whole wheat)

Instructions:
Preheat the oven to 350 degrees Fahrenheit. Combine Parmesan, garlic powder, Italian seasoning, and salt in a mixing bowl. Each pita should be cut into eight wedges and then separated into two pieces. Place on a baking sheet lined with parchment paper, and I was using a frying spray to coat the wedges. Season with the seasoning mix and bake for 10 minutes or golden brown. Allow cooling on the rack.
Nutritional Information:
Calories: 120 kcal, protein: 4 g, carbohydrates: 20 g, Fat: 3 g, Cholesterol: 2 mg, Fiber: 9 g

Sweet carrots

Preparation time: 10 minutes/**Cooking Time:** 0 minutes /**Total time:** 10 minutes
Servings: 4/**Difficulty Level:** Easy
Ingredients
- 1/4 teaspoon of salt
- 1/2 cup of water
- 1 teaspoon of trans-free margarine
- cups of shredded carrots
- The sugar substitute, to taste
- tablespoons of chopped fresh parsley,
- 1 teaspoon of lemon juice

Instructions
Boil water in a small saucepan. Add the shredded carrots and salt. Cook, after covering it, for approximately 5 minutes, or until the water has evaporated. Take the carrots off the heat. Combine the lemon juice, sugar replacement, margarine, and parsley in a large mixing bowl with carrots. Serve right away.
Nutritional Information:
Calories: 40 kcal, protein: 1 g, carbohydrates: 6 g, Fat: 1 g, Cholesterol: 0 mg, Fiber: 2.8 g

Tomato, Basil and Cucumber Salad

Preparation time: 10 minutes/**Cooking Time:** 0 minutes /**Total time:** 40 minutes
Servings: 4/**Difficulty Level:** Easy
Ingredients:
- 1 large cucumber seeded and sliced.
- 4 medium tomatoes, quartered.
- 1 medium red onion thinly sliced.
- ½ cup chopped fresh basil.
- tablespoons vinegar
- ½ teaspoon Dijon mustard
- 1 tablespoon extra-virgin olive oil
- ½ teaspoon black pepper; freshly ground.

Instructions:
Mix cucumber, tomatoes, red onion, and basil in a medium bowl. Mix vinegar, mustard, olive oil, and pepper in a small bowl. Pour the dressing over the vegetables and gently stir until well combined—cover and chill for at least 30 minutes before serving.
Nutritional Information:
Calories: 72 kcal, protein: 1 g, carbohydrates: 8 g, Fat: 4 g, Cholesterol: 4 mg, Fiber: 1 g

Thai 'Rice Noodle' Salad

Preparation time: 25 minutes/**Cooking Time:** 0 minutes /**Total time:** 25 minutes
Servings: 2/**Difficulty Level:** Easy
Ingredients:
- tbsp. fish sauce
- 1 tbsp. white vinegar
- tbsp. fresh lime juice
- 2 zucchinis
- 1/2 cup carrot peeled and grated.
- 1/4 cup peeled, diced, seeded cucumber.
- 1/4 cup scallions, sliced.
- 1 tbsp. Fresh cilantro leaves are finely chopped.
- 1 tbsp. Fresh mint leaves finely chopped.

Instructions:
Whisk dressing ingredients in a small bowl and set aside until serving. Use a julienne peeler to make zucchini noodles with the zucchinis. Mix the zucchini noodles with the salad dressing, and top with the grated carrot, sliced scallions, diced cucumber, fresh cilantro, and fresh mint leaves. Use green and yellow zucchinis mix to add more color and flavor to the dish. Stop peeling when you reach the seeds of the zucchinis, as they will not hold their shape.
Nutritional Information:

Calories: 79 kcal, protein: 4 g, carbohydrates: 13 g, Fat: 0 g, Cholesterol: 0 mg, Fiber: 3 g

Edamame and Avocado Dip

Preparation time: 5 minutes/**Cooking Time:** 0 minutes /**Total time:** 5 minutes
Servings: 4/**Difficulty Level:** Easy
Ingredients:
- 1 small avocado
- 12 oz. cooked edamame beans
- 1/2 onion, chopped.
- 1/2 cup low-fat Greek yogurt
- Juice of a lemon

Instructions:
Mash the avocado and edamame beans with a fork until smooth. Stir in the onions, Greek yogurt, and lemon juice. Serve immediately.
Nutritional Information:
Calories: 120 kcal, protein: 9 g, carbohydrates: 11 g, Fat: 5 g, Cholesterol: 0 mg, Fiber: 4 g

Zucchini Pizza Bites

Preparation time: 5 minutes/**Cooking Time:** 5 minutes /**Total time:** 10 minutes
Servings: 1/**Difficulty Level:** Easy
Ingredients
- tbsp. of quick marinara sauce
- olive oil spray
- slices of large zucchini; 1/4" thick, /1 medium diagonally cut zucchini.
- 1/4 cup of part-skim shredded mozzarella
- salt and pepper

Instructions
Cut zucchini into 1/4-inch-thick slices. Season both sides with pepper and salt after gently spraying with oil. Cook the zucchini for 2 minutes on each side on the broiler or the grill, and Broil for a further minute or two after topping with the cheese and sauce. (Be careful not to overcook the cheese.)
Nutritional Information:
Calories: 124.8 kcal, protein: 8.2 g, carbohydrates: 10.4 g, Fat: 5.7 g, Cholesterol: 12 mg, Fiber: 1.8 g

Tangy green beans

Preparation time: 10 minutes/**Cooking Time:** 0 minutes /**Total time:** 10 minutes

Servings: 10/**Difficulty Level:** Easy
Ingredients
- 1/3 cup of diced red bell peppers
- 1 1/2 pounds of green beans,
- 1/8 teaspoon of garlic powder
- 1 1/2 teaspoons of mustard
- 4 1/2 teaspoons of canola oil or olive oil
- 1 1/2 teaspoons of vinegar
- 4 1/2 teaspoons of water
- 1/4 teaspoon of pepper
- 1/4 teaspoon of salt

Instructions
Cook the beans and red peppers in the steamer basket over water until crisp-tender. In a small mixing dish, combine the remaining ingredients. Place the beans in a serving dish and set them aside. Toss in the dressing and stir to mix it well.
Nutritional Information:
Calories: 42 kcal, protein: 1 g, carbohydrates: 5 g, Fat: 2 g, Cholesterol: 0 mg, Fiber: 3.8 g

Corn pudding

Preparation time: 10 minutes/**Cooking Time:** 20 minutes /**Total time:** 30 minutes
Servings: 8/**Difficulty Level:** Easy
Ingredients
- 1/4 cup of maple syrup
- cups of coarse cornmeal (or polenta)
- 1/8 teaspoon of nutmeg
- 1/4 teaspoon of cinnamon
- cups of skim milk
- 1/8 teaspoon of clove
- 1/2 cup of raisins
- cups of water
- 1/8 teaspoon of ginger

Instructions
Bring milk and water to a boil in a saucepan. Stir in the cornmeal and keep whisking to eliminate any lumps. Bring it back to a spot. Then reduce heat and cover for 10 to 15 minutes, stirring occasionally.
Turn off the heat and add the rest of the ingredients. Allow 10 to 15 minutes for resting. Serve after a quick stir.
Nutritional Information:
Calories: 213 kcal, protein: 6 g, carbohydrates: 45 g, Fat: 1 g, Cholesterol: 2 mg, Fiber: 1.5 g

Chili-Lime Grilled Pineapple

Preparation time: 10 minutes/**Cooking Time:** 5 minutes /**Total time:** 15 minutes

Servings: 6/**Difficulty Level:** Easy

Ingredients

- tablespoons of brown sugar
- 1 fresh pineapple
- 1 tablespoon of olive oil
- 1 tablespoon of lime juice
- 1 tablespoon of agave nectar or honey
- Dash salt
- 1-1/2 teaspoons of chili powder

Instructions

Remove the eyes from the pineapple before peeling it. Next, remove the core and cut it lengthwise into six wedges. Mix the remaining ingredients in a small bowl until well combined. Half of the glaze is brushed on the pineapple; the rest should be saved for basting.

Grill covered pineapple for 2-4 minutes on each side over medium heat or broil it 4 inches from the fire until nicely browned, basting periodically with leftover glaze.

Nutritional Information:

Calories: 97 kcal, protein: 1 g, carbohydrates: 20 g, Fat: 2 g, Cholesterol: 0 mg, Fiber: 3 g

Crispy Garbanzo Beans

Preparation time: 10 minutes/**Cooking Time:** 50 minutes /**Total time:** 1 hour

Servings: 8/**Difficulty Level:** Easy

Ingredients

- 1 teaspoon of onion powder
- ½ teaspoon of salt
- 1 teaspoon of garlic powder / 4 cloves of garlic
- ½ teaspoon of pepper
- 1 teaspoon of dried parsley flakes
- cans of unsalted garbanzo beans (15 ounces)
- Cooking spray
- teaspoons of dried dill

Instructions

Preheat an oven to 400 degrees Fahrenheit. In a colander, drain and rinse garbanzo beans. Remove any excess water with a shake. To avoid "popping" in the oven, dry beans well with a towel. Combine pepper, salt, garlic powder, parsley, onion powder, and dill in a small bowl. Using cooking spray, lightly coat a rimmed baking sheet. Garbanzo beans should be spread out on a baking pan and gently sprayed with cooking spray. Season the beans with the seasoning mix and shake the pan to spread the spice evenly. Arrange the garbanzo beans in a single layer. Place the pan on the oven's lowest rack. For 30-40 minutes, cook it, carefully shaking and turning the pan every 10-15 minutes. When the beans are crispy

and golden brown, they are ready. Allow cooling completely before serving.

Nutritional Information:

Calories: 112 kcal, protein: 4.6 g, carbohydrates: 12.7 g, Fat: 5.4 g, Cholesterol: 0 mg, Fiber: 9 g

Veggie Dip

Preparation time: 15 minutes/**Cooking Time:** 0 minutes /**Total time:** 15 minutes

Servings: 3/**Difficulty Level:** Easy

Ingredients

- 1 tbsp. of Light Mayonnaise
- 1.5 tbsp. of Light Sour Cream
- tsp of Lemon Juice
- 1 tbsp. of Scallions; chopped
- 1 cup of Broccoli
- 1/4 tsp of Chili Powder
- 1 cup of Spinach
- 1 pinch of Fresh Nutmeg
- 1/8 tsp of Cayenne Pepper

Instructions:

Whirl (mix) all ingredients in a small mini chopper or the food processor. If you don't have a processor, finely chop everything, and mix it. Serve with a side of vegetables.

Nutritional Information:

Calories: 65 kcal, protein: 5.7 g, carbohydrates: 4 g, Fat: 0 g, Cholesterol: 3 mg, Fiber: 0 g

Lemon Rice

Preparation time: 10 minutes/**Cooking Time:** 45 minutes /**Total time:** 1 hour

Servings: 3 cups/**Difficulty Level:** Medium

Ingredients

- 1/4 teaspoon of kosher salt and add to taste.
- 1 tablespoon of coconut oil
- 1 cup of brown rice
- 1 3/4 cups of coconut water and a few extra tablespoons (or use unsalted vegetable)
- tablespoons of minced Italian parsley
- Juice and zest of 1 medium lemon; ¼ cup of juice

Instructions

After rinsing and draining the rice, boil it in a medium saucepan with salt, coconut water, and coconut oil.

Cook for 45 minutes after covering with a tight-fitting

cover and lowering the heat to a low simmer. Check only a few times while the rice cooks, particularly towards the finish. If the mixture seems to be drying out or sticking together, add more coconut water as required.

Turn off the heat. Toss in the lemon juice and zest, then fluff everything together with a fork. Cover and set aside for 10 minutes to allow flavors to meld. Add the parsley and mix well. Serve it warm.

Nutritional Information:
Calories: 154 kcal, protein: 3 g, carbohydrates: 28 g, Fat: 3 g, Cholesterol: 0 mg, Fiber: 1.3 g

Peanut butter hummus

Preparation time: 10 minutes/**Cooking Time:** 0 minutes /**Total time:** 10 minutes
Servings: 12/**Difficulty Level:** Medium
Ingredients
- 1/2 cup of powdered peanut butter
- 1 cup of water
- cups of garbanzo beans
- 1/4 cup of natural peanut butter
- 1 teaspoon of vanilla extract
- tablespoons of brown sugar

Instructions
In a food processor, combine all of the ingredients. Blend until completely smooth. Refrigerate it for up to a week before serving.
Nutritional Information:
Calories: 135 kcal, protein: 7 g, carbohydrates: 19 g, Fat: 4 g, Cholesterol: 0 mg, Fiber: 1.6 g

Reduced-Fat Sun-Dried Tomato Pesto

Preparation time: 2-3 minutes/**Cooking Time:** 7-8 minutes /**Total time:** 10 minutes/**Servings:** 8/**Difficulty Level:** Easy
Ingredients
- 1/4 cup walnuts
- 1/2 cup oil-packed sun-dried tomatoes
- 1/4 cup grated Parmesan cheese
- 1/2 teaspoon minced garlic
- tablespoons olive oil
- 1/4 teaspoon pepper

Instructions
Preheat oven to 375°F (190°C, or gas mark 5). Toast the nuts for 7 to 8 minutes; let cool. Drain the oil from the tomatoes. In a food processor, combine all

ingredients. Process until smooth.
Nutritional Information:
Calories: 82 kcal, protein: 3 g, carbohydrates:2 g, Fat: 8 g, Cholesterol: 3 mg, Fiber: 1 g

Boneless Buffalo Wings

Preparation time: 10 minutes/**Cooking Time:** 20 minutes /**Total time:** 30 minutes
Servings: 16/**Difficulty Level:** Easy

Ingredients
- 6 boneless, skinless chicken breasts
- tablespoons hot pepper sauce
- tablespoons white vinegar

Instructions
Preheat oven to 350°F (180°C, or gas mark 4). Cut the breasts into strips, about eight per breast. Place in roasting pan sprayed with nonstick vegetable oil spray and roast for 20 minutes, or until done. Mix hot pepper sauce and white vinegar. Place chicken pieces in a large bowl with a tight-sealing cover. Pour vinegar mixture over the elements and shake to coat. Remove, allowing the extra sauce to drain.
Nutritional Information:
Calories: 30 kcal, protein: 6 g, carbohydrates: 0 g, Fat: 0 g, Cholesterol: 15 mg, Fiber: 0 g

Steak Bites

Preparation time: 10 minutes/**Cooking Time:** 40 minutes /**Total time:** 5 hours
Servings: 16/**Difficulty Level:** Medium
Ingredients
- 1/2 cup Reduced-Sodium Soy Sauce
- 6 tablespoons sugar
- tablespoons sesame oil
- pounds round steak, cubed
- 1/2 cup chopped scallions
- 2 tablespoons white wine

Instructions
Combine the soy sauce, sugar, and sesame oil in a shallow bowl. Refrigerate the steak for 4 hours. Remove the meat from the marinade and set aside. Cook a steak to desired doneness in a large skillet over medium-high heat. In a medium saucepan, boil the reserved marinade over medium-high heat. Bring to a boil, then reduce to a low heat and simmer for 5 minutes. Add the cooked steak, scallions, and wine to the simmering marinade. Serve hot, with the entire contents of the saucepan transferred to a big bowl.

Nutritional Information:
Calories: 141 kcal, protein: 16 g, carbohydrates: 54 g, Fat: 5 g, Cholesterol: 33 mg, Fiber: 0 g

Turkey Cocktail Meatballs

Preparation time: 20 minutes/**Cooking Time:** 45 minutes /**Total time:** 1 hour 10 minutes/**Servings:** 15/**Difficulty Level:** Medium
Ingredients

- 1-pound ground turkey breast
- 1/4 cup egg substitute
- 3/4 cup saltine crackers, crushed
- 4 ounces' part-skim shredded mozzarella
- 1/4 cup chopped onion
- 1/2 teaspoon ground ginger
- 6 tablespoons Dijon mustard, divided
- 1 1/4 cups unsweetened pineapple juice
- 1/4 cup chopped green bell pepper
- tablespoons honey
- 1 tablespoon cornstarch
- 1/4 teaspoon onion powder

Instructions
Preheat oven to 350°F (180°C, or gas mark 4). Combine egg substitute, turkey, cracker crumbs, onion, ginger, mozzarella, and 3 tablespoons of mustard—form 30 balls out of the mixture, 1 inch (2.5 cm) each. Spray a 9 x 13-inch (23 x 33-cm) baking dish with nonstick vegetable oil spray—place meatballs in the container. Bake, uncovered, for 20 to 25 minutes, or until cooked through. Combine pineapple juice, green pepper, honey, cornstarch, onion powder, and remaining mustard in a saucepan. Bring to a boil, stirring constantly. Cook and stir until thickened. Brush meatballs with about 1/4 cup (60 ml) sauce and return to the oven for 10 minutes. Serve remaining sauce as a dip for meatballs.
Nutritional Information:
Calories: 100 kcal, protein: 10 g, carbohydrates: 9 g, Fat: 2 g, Cholesterol: 24 mg, Fiber: 0 g

Fat-Free Potato Chips

Preparation time: 10 minutes/**Cooking Time:** 15 minutes /**Total time:** 25 minutes
Servings: 8/**Difficulty Level:** Easy
Ingredients

- 4 medium potatoes
- Your choice of spices or herbs

Instructions
Peel the potatoes before slicing. If desired, season with your favorite spices or herbs. Place the sliced potatoes in a single layer on a microwave bacon tray if you have one. Cover with a spherical, hefty plastic cover that can be microwaved. Place potatoes between two microwave-safe plates if you don't have a bacon tray. Microwave for 7 to 8 minutes on high (full power). Depending on the wattage of your microwave, the cooking time may vary slightly. The sliced potatoes do not need to be turned over. By the time you finish, the plates will be hot.

Nutritional Information:
Calories: 129 kcal, protein: 3 g, carbohydrates: 29 g, Fat: 0 g, Cholesterol: 0 mg, Fiber: 3 g

Chicken and Mushroom Quesadillas

Preparation time: 20 minutes/**Cooking Time:** 20 minutes /**Total time:** 40 minutes
Servings: 12/**Difficulty Level:** Easy
Ingredients

- 1 tablespoon olive oil
- 21/2 teaspoons chili powder
- 1/2 teaspoon minced garlic
- 1 teaspoon dried oregano
- 8 ounces' mushrooms, sliced
- 1 cup chicken breast, cooked and shredded
- 2/3 cup onion, finely chopped
- 1/2 cup fresh cilantro, chopped
- 1 1/2 cups shredded low-fat Monterey jack cheese
- 16 5 1/2-inch (13.75-cm) corn tortillas

Instructions
Heat olive oil in a large skillet over medium-high heat. Add chili powder, garlic, and oregano and sauté for 1 minute. Add mushrooms and sauté for 10 minutes, or until tender. Remove from heat and stir in the chicken, onion, and cilantro. Cool for 10 minutes, then mix in the cheese. Spray olive oil on one side of 8 tortillas and place them on a baking sheet. Divide chicken mixture among tortillas, spreading to an even thickness. Top with the remaining tortillas and spray the tops with olive oil spray—Grill quesadillas for 3 minutes per side, or until heated through and golden brown. Cut into wedges to serve.
Nutritional Information:
Calories: 122 kcal, protein: 10 g, carbohydrates: 13 g, Fat: 4 g, Cholesterol: 13 mg, Fiber: 2 g

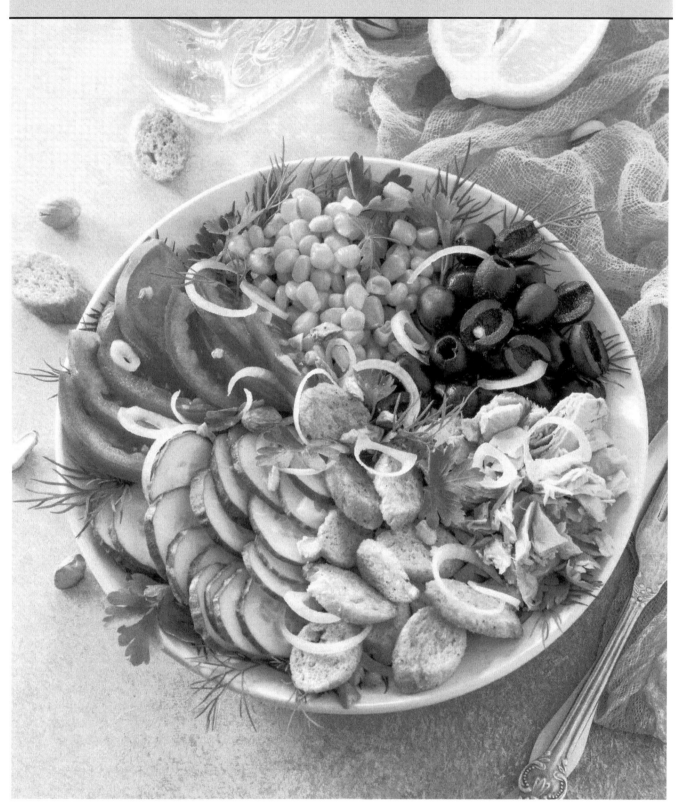

Pepper Steak Salad

Preparation time: 1-2 hours 10 minutes/**Cooking Time:** 0 minutes/**Total time:** 1-2 hours 10 minutes/**Servings:** 4/**Difficulty Level:** Easy

Ingredients:
For Marinade/Dressing:
- 1/4 cup balsamic vinegar
- 2 tablespoons sesame oil
- 1/2 teaspoon ground ginger
- 1 tablespoon sugar
- 1/4 teaspoon minced garlic
- 1-ounce sesame seeds
- 4 ounces leftover roast beef

For Salad:
- 1/2-pound lettuce, shredded
- 4 ounces snow peas
- 1/2 cup carrots, sliced
- 1 cup cabbage, shredded
- 4 ounces mushrooms, sliced
- 1/2 cup red bell pepper, sliced
- 4 ounces mung bean sprouts

Instructions:
To make the marinade/dressing:
Combine vinegar, sesame oil, ginger, sugar, garlic, and sesame seeds. Pour into a resalable plastic bag. Slice beef and add to marinade in the bag for 1 to 2 hours.

Drain, reserving liquid.

To make the salad:
Toss salad ingredients, top with beef slices. Spoon remaining dressing over.

Nutritional Information:
Calories: 216 kcal, protein: 13 g, carbohydrates: 15 g, Fat: 13 g, Cholesterol: 25 mg, Fiber: 5 g

Ambrosia with coconut and toasted almonds

Preparation time: 20 minutes/**Cooking Time:** 10 minutes/**Total time:** 30 minutes

Servings: 8/**Difficulty Level:** Easy

Ingredients
- 1 small, cubed pineapple (about 3 cups)
- 1/2 cup of shredded coconut; unsweetened
- 2 cored and diced red apples,
- 5 segmented oranges,
- 1 peeled banana halved lengthwise and sliced crosswise.
- 1/2 cup of slivered almonds
- For Garnish: Fresh mint leaves
- 2 tablespoons of cream sherry

Instructions
Set the oven to 325 degrees Fahrenheit. Spread the almonds out on a baking sheet and bake for 10 minutes, stirring periodically, until brown and fragrant. Immediately transfer to a platter to cool. Place coconut on the sheet and bake, often stirring, until the coconut is lightly toasted, for approximately 10 minutes. Immediately transfer to a platter to cool.

Combine the banana, oranges, pineapple, apples, and sherry in a large mixing bowl. Toss lightly to combine. Using separate bowls, divide the fruit mixture equally. The roasted almonds and coconut are uniformly distributed, and the mint is used as a garnish. Serve right away.

Nutritional Information:
Calories: 177 kcal, protein: 3 g, carbohydrates: 30 g, Fat: 5 g, Cholesterol: 0 mg, Fiber: 6 g

Beet walnut salad

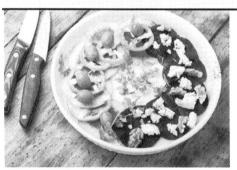

Preparation time: 20 minutes/**Cooking Time:** 0 minutes/**Total time:** 20 minutes

Servings: 8/**Difficulty Level:** Easy

Ingredients
- 1/4 cup of red wine vinegar
- 1 small bunch of beets, or canned beets (no salt added) for 3 cups, drained.
- 3 tablespoons of balsamic vinegar
- 1/4 cup of chopped celery
- 1 tablespoon of olive oil
- 1/4 cup of crumbled gorgonzola cheese,
- 8 cups of fresh salad greens

- 1 tablespoon of water
- 3 tablespoons of chopped walnuts
- 1/4 cup of chopped apple
- Freshly ground pepper.

Instructions

In a saucepan, steam raw beets in water in the saucepan until soft. Skins should be slipped off. Cool by rinsing. Using a cutter, slice it into 1/2-inch rounds. Toss with red wine vinegar in a medium mixing bowl.

Combine the olive oil, balsamic vinegar, and water in a large mixing bowl. Toss in the salad greens.

Arrange salad greens on separate salad plates. Add apples, sliced beets, and celery to the top. Pepper, cheese, and walnuts are placed over the top. Serve immediately.

Nutritional Information:

Calories: 105 kcal, protein: 3 g, carbohydrates: 12 g, Fat: 5 g, Cholesterol: 5 mg, Fiber: 3.1 g

French green lentil salad

Preparation time: 10 minutes/**Cooking Time:** 30 minutes/**Total time:** 45 minutes

Servings: 6/**Difficulty Level:** Easy

Ingredients

- 1/2 yellow finely chopped onion,
- 4 tablespoons of olive oil, divided.
- 3 minced cloves of garlic,
- 4-inch-piece of finely chopped celery stalk,
- 1 teaspoon of mustard seed
- 4-inch-piece of peeled and finely chopped carrot,
- 1 teaspoon of fennel seed
- 1/2 cup of water
- 2 cups of chicken stock or broth, vegetable stock,
- 1 bay leaf
- 1 cup of French green lentils; rinsed, picked over, then drained.
- 1/4 teaspoon of black pepper; freshly ground.
- 1 tablespoon of Dijon mustard
- 1 tablespoon of fresh chopped thyme /1 teaspoon of dried thyme
- 2 tablespoons of flat-leaf fresh (Italian) parsley, slice into strips
- 1 tablespoon of red wine vinegar or sherry vinegar

Instructions

Two teaspoons of olive oil are heated in a large saucepan over medium heat. Add and sauté the celery, onion, and carrot for approximately 5 minutes or soften the veggies. Add and sauté the mustard seed, garlic, and fennel seed for 1 minute, or until the spices are aromatic.

Add the water, stock, thyme, lentils, and bay leaf. Bring the water to a boil over medium-high heat. Reduce the heat to low, partly cover, and cook for 25 to 30 minutes, or until the lentils are cooked but firm. Drain the lentils and keep the cooking liquid aside. Remove the bay leaf and transfer the lentils to a large mixing bowl.

Combine the mustard, vinegar, and 1/4 cup of the leftover cooking liquid in a small dish. (Any leftover liquid should be discarded or saved for subsequent use.) In a separate bowl, whisk together the remaining olive oil. Toss the lentils lightly with the parsley, vinaigrette, and pepper to coat evenly. Warm the dish before serving.

Nutritional Information:

Calories: 189 kcal, protein: 11 g, carbohydrates: 25 g, Fat: 5 g, Cholesterol: 2 mg, Fiber: 3.1 g

Potato salad

Preparation time: 10 minutes/**Cooking Time:** 0 minutes/**Total time:** 10 minutes

Servings: 8/**Difficulty Level:** Easy

Ingredient

- 2 tablespoons of minced fresh dill (or 1/2 tablespoon dried)
- 1-pound potatoes, boiled and diced or steamed
- 2 ribs celery, diced (1/2 cup)
- 1 large chopped yellow onion (1 cup)
- 1/4 cup of low-calorie mayonnaise
- 1 large, diced carrot (1/2 cup)
- 1 teaspoon of ground black pepper
- 2 tablespoons of red wine vinegar
- 1 tablespoon of Dijon mustard

Instructions

In a mixing bowl, combine all ingredients and thoroughly mix them. Before serving, chill it.

Nutritional Information:

Calories: 77 kcal, protein: 1 g, carbohydrates: 2 g, Fat:

1 g, Cholesterol: 2 mg, Fiber: 1.9 g

Spinach berry salad

Preparation time: 10 minutes/**Cooking Time:** 0 minutes/**Total time:** 10 minutes

Servings: 4/**Difficulty Level:** Easy

Ingredients
- 1 cup of fresh sliced strawberries
- 4 packed cups of torn fresh spinach
- 1 cup frozen or fresh blueberries
- 1/4 cup of pecan: chopped, toasted.
- 1 small sliced sweet onion,

Salad dressing:
- 2 tablespoons of balsamic vinegar
- 1/8 teaspoon of pepper
- 2 tablespoons of honey
- 2 tablespoons of white wine vinegar or cider vinegar
- 1 teaspoon of curry powder (can be omitted)
- 2 teaspoons of Dijon mustard

Instructions
Toss onion, spinach, blueberries, strawberries, and pecans in a large salad bowl. Combine dressing ingredients in a jar with a tight-fitting cover. Shake it vigorously. Mix the salad in the dressing to coat it. Serve immediately.

Nutritional Information:
Calories: 158 kcal, protein: 4 g, carbohydrates: 25 g, Fat: 5 g, Cholesterol: 0 mg, Fiber: 2.3 g

Mexican Bean Salad

Preparation time: 10 minutes/**Cooking Time:** 0 minutes/**Total time:** 10 minutes

Servings: 8/**Difficulty Level:** Easy

Ingredients
- 2 cups cooked kidney beans
- 2 cups cooked garbanzo beans
- 1 cup tomatoes, chopped
- 3/4 cup cucumber, peeled & chopped
- 4 cups lettuce, shredded
- 1/2 cup avocado, mashed
- 2 tablespoons onion, diced
- 1/2 cup plain fat-free yogurt
- 1/4 teaspoon minced garlic

- 1/2 teaspoon cumin

Instructions
Toss together the kidney beans, garbanzo beans, tomatoes, cucumber, and onion in a large bowl. Mix the avocado, yogurt, garlic, and cumin in a small bowl. Stir the avocado mixture into the bean mixture and chill. Serve on top of shredded lettuce.

Nutritional Information:
Calories: 172 kcal, protein: 9 g, carbohydrates: 29 g, Fat: 3 g, Cholesterol: 0 mg, Fiber: 7 g

Italian Eggplant Salad

Preparation time: 2 hours 10 minutes/**Cooking Time:** 1 ½ hour/**Total time:** 3 hours 45 minutes/**Servings:** 12/**Difficulty Level:** Easy

Ingredients
- 1 crushed clove of garlic,
- 6 eggplants
- 1 tablespoon of balsamic vinegar
- ¼ teaspoon of dried basil
- 3 tablespoons of olive oil
- 1 teaspoon of dried parsley
- 2 tablespoons of white sugar
- salt and pepper to taste.
- 1 teaspoon of dried oregano

Instructions
Set the oven to 350°F (180°C) (175 degrees C). Place the eggplants on a baking sheet and pierce them with a fork. Bake for at least 1 1/2 hours, or until tender, flipping halfway through. Allow cooling before peeling and dicing. Combine the olive oil, garlic, salt, vinegar, sugar, oregano, parsley, basil, and pepper in a large mixing bowl. Stir in the chopped eggplant to coat. Allow marinating for at least 2 hours before serving.

Nutritional Information:
Calories: 95 kcal, protein: 2.4 g, carbohydrates: 15.5 g, Fat: 3.8 g, Cholesterol: 2 mg, Fiber: 3.7 g

Braised celery root

Preparation time: 10 minutes/**Cooking Time:** 10 minutes/**Total time:** 20 minutes

Servings: 6/**Difficulty Level:** Easy

Ingredients
- 1 cup of vegetable broth or stock
- 1 peeled and diced celery root (celeriac), (about 3 cups)

- 1/4 cup of sour cream
- 1 teaspoon of Dijon mustard
- 1/4 teaspoon of salt
- 1/4 teaspoon of black pepper; freshly ground.
- 2 teaspoons of fresh thyme leaves

Instructions

Boil the stock in a large saucepan over high heat. Add the celery root and mix well. Reduce the heat to low when the stock resumes to a boil. Cover and cook, occasionally turning, for 10 to 12 minutes, or until the soft celery root.

Shift the celery root to a bowl with a slotted spoon, cover, and keep warm. Raise the heat to be high and boil the cooking liquid in the saucepan. Cook, uncovered, for 5 minutes or until the liquid has been reduced to 1 tablespoon.

Whisk in the mustard, salt, sour cream, and pepper after removing the pan from the heat. Stir in the thyme and celery root until the sauce is well cooked over medium heat. Immediately transfer to a hot serving dish and serve.

Nutritional Information:

Calories: 54 kcal, protein: 2 g, carbohydrates: 7 g, Fat: 2 g, Cholesterol: 4 mg, Fiber: 2.8 g

Butternut squash and apple salad

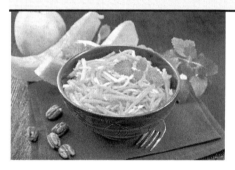

Preparation time: 10 minutes/**Cooking Time:** 30 minutes/**Total time:** 40 minutes

Servings: 6/**Difficulty Level:** Easy

Ingredients
- 2 teaspoons of olive oil
- 1 peeled and seeded, butternut squash, 1/2-inch pieces (8 cups)
- 2 large cored and sliced apples, 1/2-inch pieces
- 1 1/2 cups of chopped celery
- 6 cups of chopped spinach,
- 2 cups of chopped carrots

- 6 cups of chopped arugula,

Dressing:
- 1 1/2 teaspoons of honey
- 2 teaspoons of balsamic vinegar
- 1/2 cup of plain low-fat yogurt

Instructions

Preheat the oven to 400 degrees Fahrenheit. Squash is tossed in olive oil and roasted for 20 to 30 minutes until golden brown and tender. Allow cooling completely. In a large mixing bowl, combine all of the veggies. Whisk together the vinegar, yogurt, and honey to make the dressing. Whisk until the mixture is completely smooth. Dress the salad with the dressing. Toss it and enjoy it.

Nutritional Information:

Calories: 215 kcal, protein: 5 g, carbohydrates: 42 g, Fat: 3 g, Cholesterol: 1 mg, Fiber: 4.2 g

Yellow pear and cherry tomato salad

Preparation time: 25 minutes/**Cooking Time:** 0 minutes/**Total time:** 25 minutes

Servings: 6/**Difficulty Level:** Easy

Ingredients
For the vinaigrette
- 1 tablespoon of minced shallot
- 1/4 teaspoon of salt
- 1 tablespoon of extra-virgin olive oil
- 1 1/2 cups of halved yellow pear tomatoes,
- 1/8 teaspoon of black pepper; freshly ground.
- 2 tablespoons of red wine vinegar or sherry vinegar
- 1 1/2 cups of halved orange cherry tomatoes,
- 4 fresh large basil leaves smash into slender ribbons.
- 1 1/2 cups of halved red cherry tomatoes,

Instructions

To prepare the vinaigrette, mix the shallot and vinegar in a small dish and set aside for 15 minutes. Whisk in the salt, olive oil, and pepper until thoroughly combined. Toss all of the tomatoes together in a large serving bowl or salad bowl. Stir the tomatoes in the vinaigrette, add the basil and toss lightly to coat evenly. Serve immediately.

Nutritional Information:

Calories: 47 kcal, protein: 1 g, carbohydrates: 4 g, Fat: 3 g, Cholesterol: 0 mg, Fiber: 4.2 g

Waldorf Salad with Yogurt

Preparation time: 20 minutes/**Cooking Time:** 0 minutes/**Total time:** 20 minutes

Servings: 4/**Difficulty Level:** Easy

Ingredients
- 1 tablespoon of lemon juice
- 3 cored peeled and chopped tart apples.
- 1 cup of seedless grapes
- 2 tablespoons of chopped walnuts
- 2 chopped stalks of celery,
- ¼ teaspoon of celery seed
- 2 chopped green onions,
- 3 tablespoons of apple juice
- 2 tablespoons of mayonnaise
- 1 bunch of trimmed and chopped watercress,
- 2 tablespoons of plain yogurt

Instructions
Combine the lemon juice and apples in a large mixing bowl. Toss with celery, grapes, and green onions.

Whisk the yogurt, apple juice, grapes, and celery seeds in a small bowl. Pour over the apple mixture and gently stir. Wash and dry the watercress completely. Top with a mound of apple mixture and a sprinkling of walnuts. Arrange the greens on separate salad plates.

Nutritional Information:
Calories: 180 kcal, protein: 3.2 g, carbohydrates: 26.2 g, Fat: 8.7 g, Cholesterol: 3.6 mg, Fiber: 3 g

Mandarin Almond Salad

Preparation time: 20 minutes/**Cooking Time:** 20 minutes/**Total time:** 40 minutes

Servings: 8/**Difficulty Level:** Easy

Ingredients
- 6 thinly sliced green onions,
- 2 (11 ounces) cans of mandarin oranges, drained
- ½ cup of sliced almonds
- 2 tablespoons of white sugar
- ½ cup of olive oil
- 1 rinsed, dried, chopped head romaine lettuce
-

- ¼ cup of red wine vinegar
- 1 tablespoon of white sugar
- Ground black pepper; to taste.
- ⅛ Teaspoon of red pepper flakes; crushed.

Instructions
Combine the oranges, romaine lettuce, and green onions in a large mixing dish. In a skillet over medium heat, melt 2 tablespoons of sugar with the almonds. Cook and whisk until the sugar melts and coats the almonds. Continually stir until the nuts are light brown. Place on a platter and set aside to cool for almost 10 minutes.

In a jar with a tight-fitting lid, combine olive oil, red wine vinegar, red pepper flakes, one tablespoon of sugar, and black pepper. Shake well until the sugar is completely dissolved. Toss lettuce with salad dressing just before serving. Sprinkle sugared almonds on top and transfer to a nice serving dish.

Nutritional Information:
Calories: 235 kcal, protein: 2 g, carbohydrates: 20.2 g, Fat: 16.7 g, Cholesterol: 0 mg, Fiber: 1.8 g

Broccoli Salad

Preparation time: 45 minutes/**Cooking Time:** 0 minutes/**Total time:** 45 minutes

Servings: 6 cups /**Difficulty Level:** Easy

Ingredients
- ¼ cup of red onion; chopped.
- 6 cups of fresh broccoli; chopped.
- ½ cup of pumpkin seeds
- ¾ cup of dried cranberries
- ½ cup of mayonnaise
- 2 tablespoons of flax seeds
- 2 tablespoons of raspberry vinegar
- ½ cup of chopped pecans
- 2 tablespoons of white sugar

Instructions
Toss the pumpkin seeds, broccoli, cranberries, onion, and flax seeds together in a large mixing bowl. Add the vinegar, mayonnaise, and white sugar to a mixing bowl; pour over the salad. Toss to coat evenly. Allow at least 30 minutes for chilling before serving; top with pecans

Nutritional Information:
Calories: 380 kcal, protein: 7.2 g, carbohydrates: 29.2 g, Fat: 28.4 g, Cholesterol: 7 mg, Fiber: 2 g

Avocado Watermelon Salad

Preparation time: 15 minutes/**Cooking Time:** 0 minutes/**Total time:** 15 minutes

Servings: 6 cups /**Difficulty Level:** Easy

Ingredient
- 4 cups of fresh baby spinach, torn.
- ¼ cup of walnut oil
- 4 cups of cubed watermelon
- ¼ cup of olive oil
- 2 large peeled, pitted, diced avocados -
- ½ teaspoon of sweet paprika
- 1 lime, juiced.

Instructions
In a mixing bowl, combine the spinach, watermelon, and avocados. Combine walnut oil, lime juice, olive oil, and paprika; pour over watermelon mixture. Toss to coat evenly.

Nutritional Information:
Calories: 350 kcal, protein: 3.2 g, carbohydrates: 17.7 g, Fat: 32.2 g, Cholesterol: 2.6 mg, Fiber: 2 g

Grilled chicken salad with olives and oranges

Preparation time: 10 minutes/**Cooking Time:** 10 minutes/**Total time:** 20 minutes

Servings: 4 /**Difficulty Level:** Medium

Ingredients
For the dressing:
- 4 minced garlic cloves,
- 1/2 cup of red wine vinegar
- Cracked black pepper; to taste.
- 1 tablespoon of extra-virgin olive oil
- 1 tablespoon of finely chopped celery.
- 1 tablespoon of finely chopped red onion.

For the salad:
- 2 garlic cloves
- 4 skinless, boneless chicken breasts, 4 ounce
- 8 cups of washed and dried leaf lettuce,
- 2 navels peeled and sliced oranges,
- 16 ripe large (black) olives

Instructions
Whisk together the garlic, vinegar, olive oil, celery, onion, and pepper in a small bowl to prepare the dressing. Stir to ensure that everything is equally distributed. Cover and keep refrigerated until ready to use.

Build a fire/heat a broiler or gas grill in a charcoal grill. Spray the grill rack or broiler pan gently with cooking spray away from the heat source. Put the rack 4 to 6 inches away from the heat source. Garlic cloves should be rubbed into the chicken breasts and then discarded. For at least 5 minutes, broil or grill the chicken on each side until browned and cooked through. Allow 5 minutes for the chicken to rest on a chopping board before slicing into strips.

Two cups of lettuce, 1/4 of the sliced oranges, and 4 olives are placed on 4 plates. Drizzle dressing over each dish and top with 1 chicken breast sliced into strips. Serve right away.

Nutritional Information:
Calories: 237 kcal, protein: 27 g, carbohydrates: 12 g, Fat: 9 g, Cholesterol: 49.3 mg, Fiber: 3 g

Greek salad

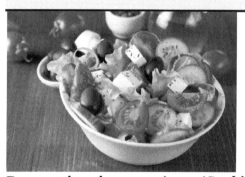

Preparation time: 20 minutes/**Cooking Time:** 20 minutes/**Total time:** 40 minutes

Servings: 8 /**Difficulty Level:** Medium

Ingredients
For the vinaigrette:
- 2 teaspoons of fresh oregano; chopped or 3/4 teaspoon of dried oregano.
- 1 tablespoon of red wine vinegar
- 1/4 teaspoon of black pepper; freshly ground.
- 1 tablespoon of fresh lemon juice
- 2 1/2 tablespoons of olive oil; extra-virgin
- 1/4 teaspoon of salt

For the salad:
- ½ diced red onion,

- 1 seeded and diced tomato,
- 1 large, trimmed eggplant, about 1 1/2 pounds, 1/2-inch cubes (about 7 cups)
- 2 tablespoons of pitted, black Greek olives; chopped.
- 1-pound stemmed spinach, torn into the bite-sized pieces
- 2 tablespoons of feta cheese; crumbled.
- 1 seeded unpeeled, and diced English (hothouse) cucumber,

Instructions

Preheat the oven to 450 degrees Fahrenheit and place a rack in the bottom third. Use olive oil cooking spray lightly coat a baking sheet.

Mix the lemon juice, vinegar, salt, oregano, and pepper in a small bowl to create the vinaigrette. Slowly drizzle in the olive oil while whisking until emulsified. Set it aside.

Arrange the eggplants in a single layer on the baking sheet that has been prepared. Using olive oil frying spray, coat the eggplant and roast it for 10 minutes, then for 8 to 10 minutes longer, turn the cubes and roast until softened and gently brown. Allow cooling fully before serving.

Combine the cucumber, spinach, onion, tomato, and cooled eggplant in a large mixing basin. Toss the salad gently in the vinaigrette to coat evenly and thoroughly. Distribute the salad among the dishes. Toss in the feta cheese and olives. Serve right away.

Nutritional Information:

Calories: 97 kcal, protein: 3 g, carbohydrates: 10 g, Fat: 5 g, Cholesterol: 2 mg, Fiber: 2 g

Fattoush

Preparation time: 10 minutes/**Cooking Time:** 10 minutes/**Total time:** 20 minutes/**Servings:** 8 /**Difficulty Level:** Medium

Ingredients
For the dressing:
- 3 minced garlic cloves,
- 1/4 cup of fresh lemon juice
- 1/2 teaspoon of salt
- 1 teaspoon of ground cumin
- 1/2 teaspoon of red pepper flakes
- 1 teaspoon of ground sumac (or lemon zest to taste)
- 2 tablespoons of olive oil; extra-virgin

- 1/4 teaspoon of black pepper; freshly ground.

For the salad:
- 3 chopped green onions with tender green tops,
- 1 chopped head of romaine lettuce (about 4 cups)
- 1 tablespoon of chopped fresh mint.
- 2 (inches in diameter) whole-wheat pitas,
- 1 seeded and diced red bell pepper,
- 2 seeded and diced tomatoes,
- 1/4 cup of fresh flat-leaf (Italian) parsley; chopped.
- 2 seeded, peeled, and diced small cucumbers,

Instructions

Make the dressing first. In a blender or food processor, combine the garlic, lemon juice, cumin, sumac (or lemon zest), red pepper flakes, salt, and black pepper. Blend until completely smooth. Slowly drizzle in the olive oil in a fine mist while the motor is running until emulsified. Place it aside.

After that, make the pita croutons. Preheat the oven to 400 degrees Fahrenheit. Rip each pita into half-inch pieces (or you may cut each into 8 triangles). Place the pieces on a baking sheet in a single layer and bake for 8 minutes, or until crisp and faintly brown. Allow cooling before serving.Now it's time to put the salad together. Toss the tomatoes, lettuce, cucumbers, green onions, mint, bell pepper, and parsley in a large mixing bowl. Toss in the dressing gently to coat evenly. Distribute the salad among the dishes. Add the croutons on top.

Nutritional Information:

Calories: 108 kcal, protein: 3 g, carbohydrates: 15 g, Fat: 4 g, Cholesterol: 0 mg, Fiber: 3.7 g

English cucumber salad with balsamic vinaigrette

Preparation time: 15 minutes/**Cooking Time:** 0 minutes/**Total time:** 15 minutes

Servings: 4 /**Difficulty Level:** Easy

Ingredient
- Cracked black pepper, to taste.
- 1 English cucumber washed and thinly sliced, with peel (8 to 9 inches in length),

For the dressing:
- 2 tablespoons of balsamic vinegar

- 1 tablespoon of fresh rosemary; finely chopped.
- 1 tablespoon of Dijon mustard
- 1 1/2 tablespoons of olive oil

Instructions

Combine the vinegar, rosemary, and olive oil in a small saucepan. Heat for 5 minutes over very low heat to combine and enhance the flavors. Remove the pan from the heat and whisk in the mustard until smooth.

Place the cucumber slices in a serving dish. Toss the cucumbers in the dressing to evenly coat them. Toss in a pinch of black pepper to taste. Place in the refrigerator until ready to serve.

Nutritional Information:

Calories: 67 kcal, protein: 0.5 g, carbohydrates: 5 g, Fat: 5 g, Cholesterol: 0 mg, Fiber: 1 g

Couscous salad

Preparation time: 10 minutes/**Cooking Time:** 0 minutes/**Total time:** 10 minutes

Servings: 8 /**Difficulty Level:** Easy

Ingredients

- 1/2 teaspoon of ground black pepper
- 1 red medium bell pepper, 1/4-inch pieces
- 1 cup of zucchini, 1/4-inch pieces
- 1/2 cup of red onion; finely chopped.
- 3/4 teaspoon of ground cumin
- 1 cup of whole-wheat couscous
- 2 tablespoons of olive oil; extra virgin
- Chopped fresh basil, parsley, or oregano for garnish (optional)
- 1 tablespoon of lemon juice

Instructions

Cook the couscous according to the package's directions. When the couscous is done, fluff it up with a fork. Add bell pepper, zucchini, cumin, onion, and black pepper. Put it aside.

Whisk together the lemon juice and olive oil in a small bowl. Toss the couscous mixture to mix. Cover and store in the refrigerator. Chill before serving. Fresh herbs may be used as a garnish.

Nutritional Information:

Calories: 136 kcal, protein: 4 g, carbohydrates: 21 g, Fat: 4 g, Cholesterol: trace, Fiber: 7 g

Artichokes alla Romana

Preparation time: 15 minutes/**Cooking Time:** 50 minutes/**Total time:** 1 hour 5 minutes/**Servings:** 8 /**Difficulty Level:** Medium

Ingredients

- 1 tablespoon of olive oil
- 2 cups of fresh whole-wheat breadcrumbs,
- 1 teaspoon of fresh oregano; chopped.
- 4 artichokes; large globe
- 1/3 cup of grated Parmesan cheese
- 2 halved lemons,
- 1 cup of dry white wine
- 3 finely chopped garlic cloves,
- 1 tablespoon of grated lemon zest
- 2 tablespoons of fresh flat-leaf finely chopped (Italian) parsley.
- 1 cup and 2 to 4 tablespoons of low-sodium chicken stock or vegetable
- 1 tablespoon of minced shallot
- 1/4 teaspoon of black pepper; freshly ground.

Instructions

Set the oven to 400 degrees Fahrenheit. Combine the olive oil and breadcrumbs in a mixing dish. Toss to coat evenly. Place the crumbs in a baking pan bake it until gently brown for approximately 10 minutes, stirring once halfway through. Allow cooling before serving.

Snip off tough outer leaves and cut the stem flush with the base, one artichoke at a time. The top third of the leaves are cut off with a serrated knife, and scissors remove any remaining thorns. To avoid discoloration, rub the sliced edges with half of a lemon. Remove the tiny leaves from the middle and separate the inner leaves. Scoop out the fuzzy choke using a spoon or melon baller, then pour some lemon juice into the hollow. Trim the rest of the artichokes the same way.

Stir the breadcrumbs with parsley, Parmesan, lemon zest, garlic, and pepper in a large mixing bowl. Add the 2 to 4 tbsp. of stock, only 1 tbsp. at a time, until the stuffing begins to cling together in tiny clumps.

Make a small mound in the middle of the artichokes with 2/3 of the filling. Spread the leaves wide, beginning at the bottom, and spoon a rounded spoonful of filling at the base of each leaf. (You may prepare the artichokes up to this stage ahead of time and keep them refrigerated.)

Combine shallot, wine, 1 cup stock, and oregano in a

Dutch oven with a tight-fitting lid. (Note: If you cook the artichokes in cast iron, they will become brown.) Boil it, then turn off the heat. Arrange the artichokes in a single layer in the liquid, stems down. Cover and cook for 45 minutes, or until the outer leaves are soft (add water if necessary). Place the artichokes on a cooling rack to cool gently. Each artichoke should be quartered and served warm.

Nutritional Information:
Calories: 123 kcal, protein: 6 g, carbohydrates: 18 g, Fat: 3 g, Cholesterol: 3 mg, Fiber: 4.2 g

Apple-fennel slaw

Preparation time: 15 minutes/**Cooking Time:** 0 minutes/**Total time:** 15 minutes

Servings: 4 /**Difficulty Level:** Easy

Ingredients
- 2 grated carrots,
- 1 medium-sized thinly sliced fennel bulb,
- 2 tablespoons of raisins
- 1 large thinly sliced and cored Granny Smith apple,
- 4 lettuce leaves
- 1/2 cup of apple juice
- 1 tablespoon of olive oil
- 2 tablespoons of apple cider vinegar
- 1 teaspoon of sugar

Instructions
Put the carrots, apple, fennel, and raisins in a large mixing bowl to prepare the slaw. Sprinkle with olive oil, cover, and chill while preparing the rest of the ingredients.

Combine the apple juice and sugar in a small saucepan. Cook, occasionally stirring until the liquid has been reduced to about 1/4 cup, approximately 10 minutes. Remove from the heat and set aside to cool. Add the apple cider vinegar and mix well. Pour the apple juice mixture over the slaw and toss to blend thoroughly.

Allow cooling completely. Serve with lettuce leaves on the side.

Nutritional Information:
Calories: 124 kcal, protein: 2 g, carbohydrates: 22 g, Fat: 4 g, Cholesterol: 0 mg, Fiber: 4 g

Salmon Salad

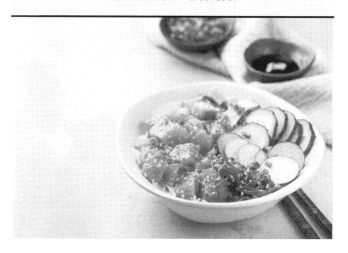

Preparation time: 10 minutes/**Cooking Time:** 0 minutes/**Total time:** 10 minutes

Servings: 4 /**Difficulty Level:** Easy

Ingredients:
- 1 diced white onion,
- 1-pound broiled salmon fillet,
- 1 cup of chopped spinach,
- 1 cup of chopped lettuce,
- 1 tablespoon of lemon juice
- 1 teaspoon of ground paprika
- 1 teaspoon of olive oil

Instructions:
Combine the onion, spinach, lettuce, salmon fillet, and paprika in a salad bowl. Shake the ingredients vigorously. The salad should then be drizzled with lemon juice and olive oil.

Nutritional Information:
Calories: 177 kcal, protein: 22.7 g, carbohydrates: 3.6 g, Fat: 8.4 g, Cholesterol: 20 mg, Fiber: 1.1 g

Grilled Vegetable Orzo Salad

Preparation time: 10 minutes/**Cooking Time:** 20 minutes/**Total time:** 30 minutes

Servings: 8/**Difficulty Level:** Medium

Ingredients:
- 1 cup zucchini, cut into 1-inch (2.5-cm) cubes
- 1/2 cup red bell pepper, cut into 1-inch (2.5-cm) cubes
- 1/2 cup yellow bell pepper, cut into 1-inch (2.5-cm) cubes
- 1 cup red onion, cut into 1-inch (2.5-cm) cubes

- 1/2 teaspoon minced garlic
- 3 tablespoons olive oil, divided
- 1 teaspoon freshly ground black pepper, divided
- 8 ounce orzo
- 1/3 cup lemon juice
- 1/4 cup pine nuts, toasted

Instructions:

Prepare the grill. Toss zucchini, bell peppers, onion, and garlic with 1 tablespoon olive oil and 1/2 teaspoon pepper in a large bowl. Transfer to a grill basket. Grill for 15 to 20 minutes, or until browned, stirring occasionally. Meanwhile, cook the orzo according to package directions. Drain and transfer to a large serving bowl. Add the roasted vegetables to the pasta. Combine the lemon juice and remaining olive oil and pepper and pour on the pasta and vegetables. Let cool to room temperature. Stir in the pine nuts

Nutritional Information:

Calories: 201 kcal, protein: 5 g, carbohydrates: 27 g, Fat: 9 g, Cholesterol: 0 mg, Fiber: 2 g

Tofu Salad

Preparation time: 10 minutes/**Cooking Time:** 0 minutes/**Total time:** 10 minutes

Servings: 6/**Difficulty Level:** Easy

Ingredients:
For Salad:
- 1/2-pound lettuce, shredded
- 4 ounces snow peas
- 1/2 cup carrot, shredded
- 1 cup cabbage, shredded
- 1/2 cup mushrooms, sliced
- 1/2 cup red bell pepper, sliced
- 4 ounces' mung bean sprouts
- 1/2 cup tomato, sliced
- 12 ounces tofu, drained and cubed
For Dressing:
- 1 tablespoon rice vinegar
- 2 tablespoons sesame oil
- 3 tablespoons Reduced-Sodium Soy Sauce
- 2 cloves garlic, crushed
- 1 tablespoon sesame seeds
- 1/2 teaspoon ground ginger

Instructions:

To make the salad: Toss salad ingredients.

To make the dressing: Combine dressing ingredients and spoon dressing over salad.

Nutritional Information:

Calories: 111 kcal, protein: 5 g, carbohydrates: 57 g, Fat: 6 g, Cholesterol: 0 mg, Fiber: 3 g

Fruited Pistachios Millet Salad

Preparation time: 10 minutes/**Cooking Time:** 15 minutes/**Total time:** 25 minutes

Servings: 4/**Difficulty Level:** Easy

Ingredients:
- 1 cup millet
- ½ cup pistachios, toasted
- ½ cup dried longings
- ½ cup peanuts, toasted
- 2 kiwifruits, diced
- Zest and juice of 2 orange
- 3 tbsps. ruby port
- 2 tbsps. finely chopped turmeric

Instructions:

Bring 2 quarts of lightly salted water to a boil over high heat and pour the millet. Return to a boil, lower the heat to medium, cover, and simmer for 12 to 14 minutes. Drain off the water, rinse millet until cool, set aside. Whisk the orange juice, zest, and ruby port in a large bowl. Toss until well combined. Stir in the pistachios, longings, peanuts, kiwifruit, and turmeric and toss until well combined. Put in the cooked millet and toss to blend. Refrigerate before serving.

Nutritional Information:

Calories: 388 kcal, protein: 7.8 g, carbohydrates: 87.2 g, Fat: 31.3 g, Cholesterol: 0 mg, Fiber: 8.3 g

Lemony Kale Salad

Preparation time: 10 minutes/**Cooking Time:** 10 minutes/**Total time:** 20 minutes

Servings: 4/**Difficulty Level:** Easy

Ingredients:
- 2 heads kale
- Sea salt and freshly ground pepper
- Juice of 1 lemon
- 1 tbsp. olive oil
- 2 cloves garlic, minced
- 1 cup cherry tomatoes, sliced

Instructions:

Wash and dry kale. Tear the kale into small pieces. Heat olive oil in a large skillet and add the garlic. Cook for 1 minute and then add the kale. Add the tomatoes after kale wilted. Cook until tomatoes are softened, then remove from heat. Put tomatoes and kale together in a bowl, and season with sea salt and freshly ground pepper. Drizzle with remaining olive oil and lemon juice, serve.

Nutritional Information:
Calories: 59 kcal, protein: 2 g, carbohydrates: 5.95 g, Fat: 3.83g, Cholesterol: 0 mg, Fiber: 1.9 g

Rice Noodle Zucchini Salad with Tuna

Preparation time: 25 minutes/**Cooking Time:** 0 minutes/**Total time:** 25 minutes

Servings: 4/**Difficulty Level:** Easy

Ingredients:
- 4 cups cooked rice vermicelli
- 4 zucchinis, peeled into long ribbons with a vegetable peeler
- 2 cups shredded carrot
- 2 (5-ounce) can chunk albacore tuna, drained
- ½ cup store-bought sesame dressing

Instructions:
Toss together the noodles, zucchini, carrot, and tuna in a large bowl. Add the dressing and toss to coat before serving.

Nutritional Information:
Calories: 405 kcal, protein: 19 g, carbohydrates: 50 g, Fat: 15 g, Cholesterol: 25 mg, Fiber: 5 g

Succotash Salad with Peanut Butter

Preparation time: 10 minutes/**Cooking Time:** 0 minutes/**Total time:** 10 minutes

Servings: 4/**Difficulty Level:** Easy

Ingredients:
- 1½ cups cooked fava beans
- 3 ears corn, shucked (about 2 cups)
- 2 large avocados, peeled and diced
- 1 medium zucchini, peeled and diced
- ¼ cup (60mL) peanut butter
- ¼ cup chopped basil
- Salt and freshly ground black pepper to taste

Instructions:
Mix all the ingredients in a large bowl and toss to combine well.

Nutritional Information:
Calories: 177 kcal, protein: 8.63 g, carbohydrates: 35.58 g, Fat: 1.26 g, Cholesterol: 0 mg, Fiber: 8.2 g

Spinach Quinoa Salad with Pomegranate Citrus Dressing

Preparation time: 15 minutes/**Cooking Time:** 15 minutes/**Total time:** 30 minutes

Servings: 6/**Difficulty Level:** Medium

Ingredients:
- 1 cup extra-virgin olive oil
- 3 cups baby spinach
- 1½ cups water
- 1 cup quinoa
- ¼ tsp. kosher salt
- ½ cup pomegranate juice
- ½ cup freshly squeezed orange juice
- 1 small shallot, minced
- 1 tsp. pure maple syrup
- 1 tsp. za'atar
- ½ tsp. ground sumac
- ½ tsp. kosher salt
- ¼ tsp. freshly ground black pepper
- ½ cup fresh parsley, coarsely chopped
- ½ cup fresh mint, coarsely chopped
- Approximately ¾ cup pomegranate seeds, or 2 pomegranates
- ¼ cup pistachios shelled and toasted
- ¼ cup crumbled blue cheese

Instructions:
To make the quinoa: Bring the water, quinoa, and salt to a boil in a small saucepan. Reduce the heat and cover, simmer for 10 to 12 minutes. Fluff with a fork.

To Make the Dressing: Whisk together the olive oil, pomegranate juice, orange juice, shallot, maple syrup, za'atar, sumac, salt, and black pepper in a medium bowl. In a separate large bowl, add about ½ cup of dressing. Store the remaining dressing in a glass jar or airtight container and refrigerate. The dressing can be kept for up to 2 weeks. Let the chilled dressing reach room temperature before using.

To make the salad: Combine the spinach, parsley, and

mint in the bowl with the dressing and toss gently together. Add the quinoa and toss gently, then add the pomegranate seeds. If using whole pomegranates: Cut the pomegranates in half. Fill a large bowl with water and hold the pomegranate in half, cut-side-down. Using a wooden spoon, hit the back of the pomegranate, so the seeds fall into the water. Immerse the pomegranate in the water and gently pull out any remaining seeds. Repeat with the remaining pomegranate. Skim the white pith off the top of the water. Drain the seeds and add them to the greens. Add the pistachios and cheese and toss gently.

Nutritional Information:
Calories: 300 kcal, protein: 8 g, carbohydrates: 28 g, Fat: 19 g, Cholesterol: 6 mg, Fiber: 5 g

Tomato Pasta Salad

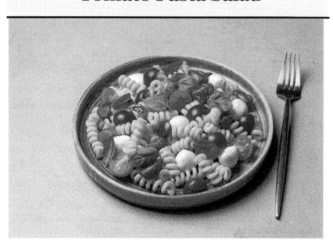

Preparation time: 10 minutes/**Cooking Time:** 20 minutes/**Total time:** 1 hour 30 minutes/**Servings:** 8/**Difficulty Level:** Medium

Ingredients:
- 2 cups dried pasta
- 1 cup fat-free sour cream
- 1/4 cup skim milk
- 1 tablespoon fresh dill
- 1 tablespoon vinegar
- 1/2 teaspoon black pepper
- 2 cups cucumber, chopped
- 2 cups tomatoes, chopped

Instructions:
Cook pasta in boiling salted water until al dente. Drain and rinse in cold water. Transfer cooked pasta to a large serving bowl. Mix sour cream, milk, dill, vinegar, and pepper separately. Set dressing aside. Mix cucumbers and tomatoes into the pasta. Pour dressing over pasta mixture and toss thoroughly to combine.

Cover, and refrigerate for at least 1 hour and preferably overnight. Stir just before serving.

Nutritional Information:
Calories: 91 kcal, protein: 3 g, carbohydrates: 11 g, Fat: 1 g, Cholesterol: 19 mg, Fiber: 1 g

Garbanzo and Pasta Salad

Preparation time: 10 minutes/**Cooking Time:** 0 minutes/**Total time:** 8 hours 10 minutes/**Servings:** 8/**Difficulty Level:** Easy

Ingredients:
- 4 ounces' pasta
- 2 cups cooked garbanzo beans
- 1/2 cup red bell pepper, chopped
- 113 cup celery, sliced
- 113 cup carrot, sliced
- 1/4 cup scallions, chopped
- 3 tablespoons balsamic vinegar
- 2 tablespoons low-fat mayonnaise
- 2 teaspoons mustard
- 1/2 teaspoon black pepper
- 1/4 teaspoon dried Italian seasoning
- 4 cups leaf lettuce, torn into bite-sized pieces

Instructions:
Cook pasta according to directions, omitting salt. Drain and rinse well under cold water until pasta is cool; drain well. Combine pasta, garbanzo beans, red bell pepper, celery, carrot, and scallions in a medium bowl. Whisk together vinegar, mayonnaise, mustard, black pepper, and Italian seasoning in a small bowl until blended. Pour over salad; toss to coat evenly. Cover and refrigerate for up to 8 hours. Arrange lettuce on individual plates. Spoon salad over lettuce.

Nutritional Information:
Calories: 150 kcal, protein: 6 g, carbohydrates: 26 g, Fat: 3 g, Cholesterol: 13 mg, Fiber: 4 g

Coleslaw

Preparation time: 10 minutes/**Cooking Time:** 0 minutes/**Total time:** 10 minutes
Servings: 6/**Difficulty Level:** Easy

Ingredients:
- 2 cups cabbage, shredded
- 113 cup carrot, shredded
- 1/4 cup low-fat mayonnaise
- 1/4 cup fat-free sour cream
- 2 tablespoons vinegar

- 2 tablespoons sugar
- 1/4 teaspoon celery seed
- 1/4 teaspoon onion powder

Instructions:
Stir dressing ingredients together. Pour over cabbage and stir to mix.

Nutritional Information:
Calories: 75 kcal, protein: 1 g, carbohydrates: 8 g, Fat: 3 g, Cholesterol: 7 mg, Fiber: 1 g

Roasted Corn Salad

Preparation time: 10 minutes/**Cooking Time:** 0 minutes/**Total time:** 2 hours 10 minutes/**Servings:** 4/**Difficulty Level:** Easy

Ingredients:
- 4 ears of corn
- 1/4 cup red bell pepper, chopped
- 1/4 cup onion, chopped
- 2 tablespoons honey
- 1/4 cup lime juice
- 1 tablespoon fresh coriander
- 1/4 teaspoon cumin

Instructions:
Husk and clean corn. Wrap in aluminum foil. Grill over medium heat until tender, turning often. Cut corn from cobs. Stir in pepper and onion. Mix remaining ingredients. Pour over vegetables. Stir to mix. Refrigerate at least 2 hours or overnight before serving.

Nutritional Information:
Calories: 101 kcal, protein: 2 g, carbohydrates: 26 g, Fat: 0 g, Cholesterol: 0 mg, Fiber: 2 g

Black Bean Salad

Preparation time: 40 minutes/**Cooking Time:** 2 hours /**Total time:** 2 hours 40 minutes/**Servings:** 8/**Difficulty Level:** Easy

Ingredients:
- 3/4 cup dried black beans
- 3/4 cup dried black-eyed peas
- 1 cup onion, chopped
- 2 cups smoked turkey breast
- 1 cup low-fat Italian salad dressing
- 1 cup scallions, chopped
- 1 1/3 cups red bell pepper, chopped
- 1 1/4 cups frozen corn, thawed
- 1/4 cup cilantro, chopped
- 2 teaspoons curry powder
- 1/2 teaspoon red pepper flakes

Instructions:
Place beans and peas in separate saucepans. Cover with water. Add half of the onion to each. Bring to a boil and boil for 1 minute. Remove from heat, cover, and let stand for 1 hour. Add additional water to saucepans if needed. Divide turkey between pans. Simmer for one hour or until beans are tender. Drain. Combine beans, black-eyed peas, and turkey in a large bowl. Pour Italian dressing over while hot. Add scallions, red bell pepper, corn, cilantro, curry powder, and red pepper flakes. Toss to mix. Cover and refrigerate overnight or serve warm.

Nutritional Information:
Calories: 161 kcal, protein: 15 g, carbohydrates: 19 g, Fat: 4 g, Cholesterol: 26 mg, Fiber: 4 g

Asian-Style Chicken Salad

Preparation time: 10 minutes plus marination time/**Cooking Time:** 0 minutes

Total time: 10 minutes /**Servings:** 4/**Difficulty Level:** Easy

Ingredients:
- 6 cups iceberg lettuce, torn into bite-sized pieces
- 1/4 cup scallions, sliced
- 1/2 cup cilantro, chopped
- 1/2 cup fresh parsley, chopped
- 1/2 cup celery, sliced
- 1/4 cup rice vinegar
- 1 tablespoon sesame oil
- 1/4 cup Reduced-Sodium Soy Sauce
- 1 tablespoon sesame seeds
- 2 cups cooked chicken breast, chopped
- 1/2 cup mandarin oranges
- 1/4 cup slivered almonds

Instructions:
Chop lettuce, scallions, cilantro, parsley, and celery and toss together. Combine vinegar, sesame oil, soy sauce, and sesame seeds for dressing. Marinate the chopped chicken in the dressing for a few hours or

overnight. Before serving, add oranges, almonds, and chicken with dressing to the salad. Toss well.

Nutritional Information:
Calories: 247 kcal, protein: 25 g, carbohydrates: 108 g, Fat: 11 g, Cholesterol: 60 mg, Fiber:

Pork Salad

Preparation time: 10 minutes plus marination time/**Cooking Time:** 20 minutes

Total time: 1-2 hours 30 minutes /**Servings:** 6/**Difficulty Level:** Easy

Ingredients:
For Marinade
- 4 boneless pork loin chops
- 1/4 cup Reduced-Sodium Soy Sauce (see recipe page 30)
- 1 tablespoon sesame oil
- 1 tablespoon rice vinegar
- 1 tablespoon sugar

For Salad:
- 1/2-pound lettuce, shredded
- 4 ounces snow peas
- 1/2 cup carrot, sliced
- 1 cup cabbage, shredded
- 4 ounces mushrooms, sliced
- 1/2 cup red bell pepper, sliced
- 4 ounces mung bean sprouts

For Dressing:
- 1/4 cup Reduced-Sodium Soy Sauce
- 2 tablespoons rice vinegar
- 2 tablespoons mirin wine
- 1/2 teaspoon ground ginger
- 1 tablespoon sesame seeds

Instructions:
Thinly slice chops. Combine soy sauce, sesame oil, vinegar, and sugar. Place pork and marinade in a resealable plastic bag and marinate for 1 to 2 hours. Drain and stir-fry until cooked through. Toss salad ingredients, top with pork slices. Combine all dressing ingredients and spoon dressing over salad to serve.

Nutritional Information:
Calories: 173 kcal, protein: 17 g, carbohydrates: 140 g, Fat: 5 g, Cholesterol: 42 mg, Fiber: 2 g

Steak salad with roasted corn vinaigrette

Preparation time: 5 minutes /**Cooking Time:** 20 minutes/**Total time:** 25 minutes

Servings: 6/**Difficulty Level:** Easy

Ingredients
- 2 tablespoons of fresh lime juice
- 1/2 cup of water
- 2 tablespoons of extra-virgin olive oil
- 3 cups of fresh corn kernels / frozen corn kernels, thawed.
- 2 tablespoons of chopped red bell pepper.
- 1/2 teaspoon of salt
- 1/4 cup of fresh chopped cilantro (fresh coriander)
- 1/2 teaspoon of black pepper; freshly ground.
- 1 tablespoon of ground cumin
- 1/4 teaspoon of red pepper flakes
- 2 teaspoons of dried oregano
- 1 large, trimmed head romaine lettuce, bite-sized pieces (about 6 cups)
- 3/4 pound of (12 ounces) flank steak
- 4 cups of halved cherry tomatoes,
- 1 1/2 cups of no salt added to cooked black beans,
- 3/4 cup of red onion; thinly sliced.

Instructions
Over medium-high heat, dry a nonstick heavy frying pan or big cast iron. Add and cook until the corn starts to brown, often turning for about 4 to 5 minutes. Take the pan off the heat and put it aside.

Combine the bell pepper, lime juice, water, and 1 cup of roasted corn in a food processor. Pulse until smooth. Add the olive oil, 1/4 teaspoon of black pepper, 1/4 teaspoon of salt, and the cilantro in a mixing bowl. Blend using a pulsing motion. Set aside the vinaigrette.

In a charcoal grill, make a fire, or heat a broiler or gas grill. Spray the broiler pan or grill rack gently with cooking spray, away from the heat source. Place the rack 4 to 6 inches away from the heat source.

Combine the red pepper flakes, oregano, cumin, and the remaining 1/4 teaspoon of salt and 1/4 teaspoon of black pepper in a small bowl. Rub both sides of the steak with the rub. Place the steak on the broiler pan or grill rack and cook, flipping once, for 4 to 5 minutes on each side, until browned. Do you check for doneness by cutting into the middle (medium doneness is 160 F if using a meat thermometer)? Allow for a 5-minute rest period. Using a sharp knife, cut small slices across the grain. Cut the slices into 2-inch-long segments.

Combine the tomatoes, lettuce, black beans, onion, and leftover roasted corn in a large mixing bowl. Toss in the vinaigrette gently to combine and coat evenly. Divide the salad among the separate dishes to serve. Grilled steak pieces should be placed on top of each dish.

Nutritional Information:
Calories: 295 kcal, protein: 21 g, carbohydrates: 140 g, Fat: 9 g, Cholesterol: 36 mg, Fiber: 9 g

Pickled onion salad

Preparation time: 10 minutes /**Cooking Time:** 0 minutes/**Total time:** 1 hour 10 minutes/**Servings:** 4/**Difficulty Level:** Easy

Ingredients
- 4 chopped spring (green) onions with tops,
- 2 large thinly sliced red onions (about 2 cups)
- 2 teaspoons of olive oil
- 4 lettuce leaves
- 1/2 cup of cider vinegar
- 2 tablespoons of sugar
- 1 tablespoon of lime juice
- 1/2 cup of fresh chopped cilantro,

Instructions
Combine the onions, oil, vinegar, and sugar in a small bowl. Stir to ensure that everything is evenly distributed. Refrigerate for at least 60 minutes, covered and chilled. Stir in the cilantro just before serving, and season with lime juice. Serve neatly stacked on a lettuce leaf.

Nutritional Information:
Calories: 86 kcal, protein: 1 g, carbohydrates: 16 g, Fat: 2 g, Cholesterol: 0 mg, Fiber: 1 g

Grilled cod with crispy citrus salad

Preparation time: 5 minutes /**Cooking Time:** 15 minutes/**Total time:** 20 minutes

Servings: 2/**Difficulty Level:** Easy

Ingredients
- 1 teaspoon of olive oil
- 8 ounces of cod
- 1 1/2 cups of chopped spinach
- 1 cup of diced celery
- 1 1/2 cups of shredded kohlrabi
- 2 tablespoons of chopped fresh basil.
- 1 1/2 cups of shredded carrot
- 3/4 cup of red bell pepper; chopped.
- 1 tablespoon of chopped fresh parsley.
- Zest and juice of one Lemon
- 1 tablespoon of minced garlic (about 4 large cloves) or to taste.
- Zest and juice of one lime
- 1 large grapefruit (about 1 cup), cut into segments.
- Zest and juice of one orange
- Black pepper to taste.
- 1 medium orange (about 1/2 cup), cut into segments.

Instructions
Using cooking spray, coat a grill/ broiler pan. Heat the grill or the broiler. Brush lightly with oil and place fish on broiler or grill pan.

Grill or broil at 3-4 inches away from the flame for 10 minutes or until salmon flakes readily with a fork. The fish must achieve a temperature of 145 degrees Fahrenheit on the inside. Put it aside.

Toss the other ingredients in a large mixing bowl, except the orange segments and grapefruit. Salad should be divided between two dishes. Season with black pepper to taste and top with cod and citrus slices.

Nutritional Information:
Calories: 412 kcal, protein: 26 g, carbohydrates: 50 g, Fat: 12 g, Cholesterol: 47 mg, Fiber: 13

Chapter 10: Soups and Stews

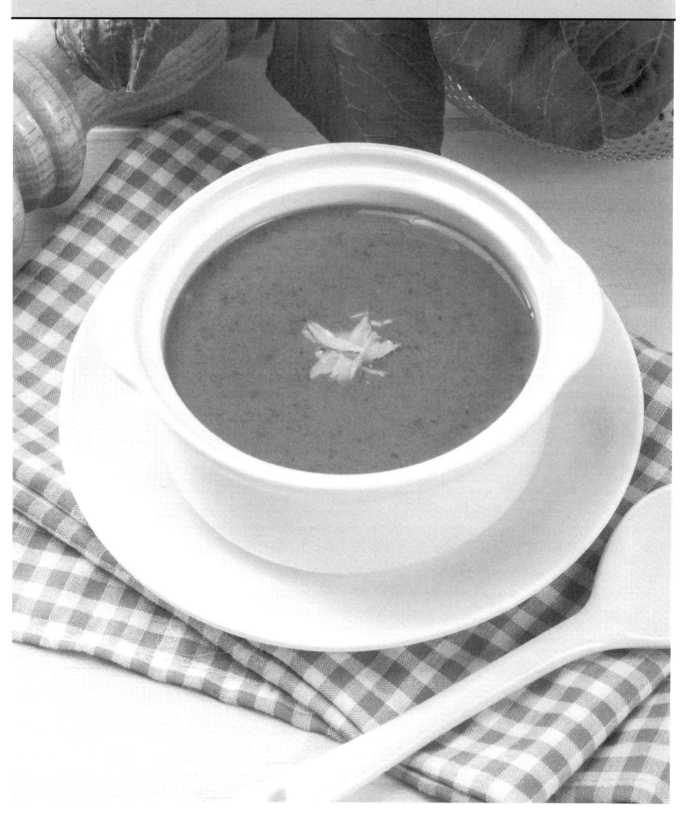

Carrot soup

Preparation time: 5 minutes/**Cooking Time:** 25 minutes/**Total time:** 30 minutes

Servings: 6/**Difficulty Level:** Easy

Ingredients:

- 2 cups of water
- 1 1/2 tablespoons of sugar
- 10 scraped and sliced carrots,
- 1/4 teaspoon of ground black pepper
- 3 tablespoons of plain all-purpose flour
- 1/4 teaspoon of ground nutmeg
- 2 tablespoons of fresh chopped parsley
- 4 cups of fat-free milk

Instructions

Heat the carrots, sugar, and water in a large saucepan. Cover and cook for 20 minutes, or until the carrots are soft. Drain and set aside some of the juice from the carrots. Place aside.

Whisk together flour, nutmeg, pepper, and milk in a second saucepan over medium-high heat. Cook until the white sauce thickens, stirring frequently.

Combine the white sauce and the cooked carrots in a blender or food processor. Puree until completely smooth. To get the required consistency, add the reserved liquid. Pour into individual bowls and top with 1 teaspoon of parsley. Serve immediately.

Nutritional Information: Calories: 124 kcal, protein: 7 g, carbohydrates: 24 g, Fat: traces g, Cholesterol: 3 mg, Fiber: 3.2 g

Home-style turkey soup

Preparation time: 10 minutes/**Cooking Time:** 2 hours/**Total time:** 2 hours 10 minutes/**Servings:** 10/**Difficulty Level:** Medium
Ingredients:

For the broth:

- 4 cups of water
- 1 turkey carcass
- 3 large onions;1 quartered and 3 chopped.
- 8 cups of low-sodium chicken broth

For the soup:

- 1 cup of peeled diced rutabaga or turnip,
- 1/4 cup of chopped fresh parsley.
- 1 chopped onion,
- 4 peeled carrots, thin strips
- 1 cup of chopped celery
- 1/4 cup of uncooked pearl barley
- 1/2 teaspoon of ground black pepper
- 1/4 teaspoon of dried thyme
- 1 can (16 ounces) of white beans; rinsed and drained
- 1 bay leaf
- 1/2-pound leftover bite-size chunks of light turkey meat
- 1 can (14 ounces) of unsalted tomatoes

Instructions

Combine the water, turkey carcass, broth, and quartered onion in a large stockpot. Over high heat, bring to a boil. Reduce the heat to low, cover, and cook for 1 hour. Remove the carcass and onion from the mixture and strain it. Refrigerate the liquid — preferably overnight — and skim the fat from the surface of the soup.

Toss the liquid back into the stockpot. Toss the soup ingredients into the broth. Bring to a low simmer and cook for 1 hour, covered. Immediately ladle into separate bowls and serve.

Nutritional Information: Calories: 178 kcal, protein: 15 g, carbohydrates: 25 g, Fat:2 g, Cholesterol: 23 mg, Fiber: 5 g

Pea Soup

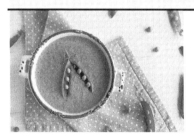

Preparation time: 10 minutes/**Cooking Time:** 3 hours/**Total time:** 3 hours 10 minutes

Servings: 16/**Difficulty Level:** Medium

Ingredients:

- 1 meaty ham bone
- 1/2 pound of dried whole peas
- 3 quarts of water
- 1/2 pound of dried green split peas
- 2 chopped celery ribs,
- 1 large, chopped onion,
- 1/2 cup of chopped celery leaves
- 1 tablespoon of minced fresh parsley
- 1/2 pound of chopped, smoked sausage, optional.
- 1 medium chopped carrot,
- 1 teaspoon of salt
- 1 teaspoon of bouquet garni (mixed herbs)
- 1/4 teaspoon of pepper
- 1 bay leaf

Spaetzle Dumplings:

- 1 large beaten egg,
- 1/3 cup of water
- 1 cup of all-purpose flour

Instructions

Soak peas overnight, covered with water. Place in a Dutch oven after draining and rinsing. Except for the sausage and dumplings, add the water, ham bone, and the other soup ingredients. Bring the water to a boil. Reduce the heat to low, cover, and cook for 2 to 2-1/2 hours.

Remove the ham bone and any excess fat. Pull the flesh off the bone and dice it. Toss in the ham and, if wanted, the sausage to the pan. Fill a small bowl halfway with flour for dumplings. Make a hole in the middle of the flour and pour in the egg and water, stirring until smooth.

Place a 3/16-inch-diameter-holed colander over the boiling soup; transfer the dough to the colander and push it through with a wooden spoon. Cook for 10-15 minutes, uncovered. Bay leaf should be discarded. Option to Freeze: Make the soup without the dumplings and freeze it in serving-size quantities to enjoy for months.

Nutritional Information:

Calories: 155 kcal, protein: 9 g, carbohydrates: 26 g, Fat:2 g, Cholesterol: 20 mg, Fiber: 4.1 g

Three Sisters Soup

Preparation time: 5 minutes/**Cooking Time:** 40 minutes/**Total time:** 45 minutes

Servings: 6/**Difficulty Level:** Medium

Ingredients:

- 16 oz. Low-sodium canned of yellow corn or hominy drained and rinsed.
- 6 cups of low-sodium fat-free, chicken or vegetable stock
- 1/2 tsp. of curry powder
- 16 oz. low-sodium canned of kidney beans (drained, rinsed)
- 15 oz. of cooked, canned pumpkin
- 1 small, chopped onion.
- 5 fresh sage leaves OR 1/2 tsp. of dried sage
- 1 chopped rib celery

Instructions

Bring the chicken stock to a boil. Corn/hominy, onion, beans, and celery are added. Boil for 10 minutes at a low temperature. Simmer for 20 minutes over medium-low heat with curry, sage leaves, and pumpkin.

Nutritional Information: Calories: 145 kcal, protein: 9 g, carbohydrates: 28 g, Fat:1 g, Cholesterol: 0 mg, Fiber: 6 g

Fish Stew with Tomatoes

Preparation time: 5 minutes/**Cooking Time:** 40 minutes/**Total time:** 45 minutes

Servings: 4/**Difficulty Level:** Medium

Ingredients:

- 1 medium chopped green bell pepper
- 1 tsp. of canola or corn oil
- 1/2 medium chopped onion
- 3 thin white fish fillets; catfish or tilapia (4 ounces each), patted dry, rinsed, one-inch cubes.
- 1 medium chopped carrot (quartered lengthwise)
- 1 cup of water

- 14.5 oz. of no-salt-added, canned, diced tomatoes (undrained)
- 1 tsp. of salt-free Creole or Cajun seasoning blend
- 1 ounce of baking potatoes (peeled, diced)
- 1/2 tsp. of salt
- 2 teaspoon of light tub margarine

Instructions

Heat the oil in a Dutch oven over medium-high heat, stirring it to coat the bottom. Add and cook the carrot, bell pepper, and onion for 3 minutes, stirring often, or until the onion is tender. Add the potato, tomatoes, water, liquid, and spice blend. Bring the water to a boil. Reduce the heat to low and cover the saucepan for 20 minutes, or until the potatoes are cooked.

Stir in the fish gently. Cook for 5 minutes, covered, or until the fish readily flakes when checked with a fork. Turn off the heat.

Fold in the margarine and salt gently so that the fish does not break apart. Allow approximately 5 minutes of resting time, covered, to allow the flavors to blend. Pour the soup into soup bowls.

Nutritional Information:

Calories: 172 kcal, protein: 19 g, carbohydrates: 16 g, Fat:3.5 g, Cholesterol: 36 mg, Fiber: 2.2 g

Vegetable, lentil, and garbanzo bean stew

Preparation time: 10 minutes/**Cooking Time:** 7 hours 40 minutes/**Total time:** 8 hours

Servings: 8/**Difficulty Level:** Medium

Ingredients:

- 4 cups of vegetable stock; low-sodium
- 3 cups of butternut squash (1 1/2 -2 pounds), seeded, peeled, 1-inch cubes.
- 2 large, chopped onions,
- 3 large, peeled carrots, 1/2-inch pieces
- 1 cup of red lentils
- 3 minced garlic cloves,
- 1/4 teaspoon of saffron
- 2 tablespoons of tomato paste; no-added-salt

- 1 teaspoon of turmeric
- 2 teaspoons of ground cumin
- 1/4 cup of lemon juice
- 1/2 cup of fresh chopped Cilantro
- 2 tablespoons of peeled, minced fresh ginger.
- 1 teaspoon of freshly ground pepper.
- 1/2 cup of chopped unsalted roasted peanuts.
- 1 can (16 ounces) of garbanzo beans; drained and rinsed.

Instructions

Slowly cook veggies (squash, onions, carrots, and garlic) in a Dutch oven over low-medium heat until onions turn brown. Scrape up the browned pieces of veggies from the bottom of the pan with the vegetable stock.

Add the tomato paste, lentils, and seasonings. Cover and simmer over medium-low heat for 1 to 1 1/2 hours, or until lentils and squash are tender. Stir once in a while. Alternatively, put the ingredients in a slow cooker and simmer on low for 4-6 hours.

Add the lemon juice and garbanzo beans. Serve hot with chopped peanuts and cilantro on top.

Nutritional Information: Calories: 287 kcal, protein: 13 g, carbohydrates: 41 g, Fat: 7 g, Cholesterol: 0 mg, Fiber: 9 g

Zesty tomato soup

Preparation time: 5 minutes/**Cooking Time:** 15 minutes/**Total time:** 20 minutes

Servings: 2/**Difficulty Level:** Easy

Ingredients:

- 2 tablespoons of croutons
- 1 can (10.5 ounces) of condensed low-fat, low-sodium, tomato soup
- 1 medium chopped tomato,
- 1 can of (10.5 ounces) fat-free milk
- 1 tablespoon of Parmesan cheese; freshly grated.
- 1 tablespoon of fresh chopped basil or Cilantro

Instructions

Combine the soup and milk in a saucepan. Whisk it together until it's completely smooth. Warm for 7 to 10 minutes over medium heat, stirring regularly. Add the chopped herbs and tomato. Cook for 5 minutes more, stirring periodically.

Pour evenly into individual bowls and top with 1 tablespoon of croutons and 1 1/2 teaspoons of Parmesan cheese. Serve immediately.

Nutritional Information:

Calories: 178 kcal, protein: 9 g, carbohydrates: 31 g, Fat: 2 g, Cholesterol: 5 mg, Fiber: 9 g

Quibebe soup

Preparation time: 5 minutes/**Cooking Time:** 35 minutes/**Total time:** 40 minutes

Servings: 8/**Difficulty Level:** Easy

Ingredients:

- 2 cups of chopped onions
- 1 tablespoon of olive oil
- 2 chopped Fresno chili peppers,
- 1 1/2 cups of diced tomatoes
- 8 cups of vegetable stock; low-sodium
- 1 1/2 diced garlic cloves,
- 3/4 teaspoon of salt
- 1 cubed butternut squash,
- 2 1/2 tablespoons of chopped fresh parsley.
- 1/2 teaspoon of sugar
- 3/4 teaspoon of ground black pepper

Instructions

Add the oil to a large stockpot over medium heat. Add and cook Fresno peppers, onions, tomatoes, and garlic for approximately 15 minutes, stirring often. Add the squash and vegetable stock to the pot. Bring to a boil, then turn down the heat to low.

Once the squash is cooked (approximately 15 minutes), purée the soup in small batches in a blender until smooth. Put the soup back in the pot. Combine the pepper, salt, and sugar in a mixing bowl. Before serving, garnish with parsley.

Nutritional Information: Calories: 106 kcal, protein: 2 g, carbohydrates: 12 g, Fat: 4 g, Cholesterol: 0 mg, Fiber: 3 g

Potato-fennel soup

Preparation time: 5 minutes/**Cooking Time:** 35 minutes/**Total time:** 30 minutes

Servings: 8/**Difficulty Level:** Easy

Ingredients:

- 3 cups of chicken broth; reduced-sodium.
- 1 cup of chopped red onion.
- 2 large peeled and sliced russet potatoes,
- 1 large, chopped fennel bulb (about 2 pounds),
- 2 teaspoons of toasted fennel seeds,
- 1 cup of fat-free milk
- 1 teaspoon of olive oil
- 2 teaspoons of lemon juice

Instructions

Heat the olive oil in a large soup pot over medium heat. Fennel and onion are added. Cook for approximately 5 minutes or until the veggies are tender. Add the potatoes, milk, chicken broth, and lemon juice. Cover, lower the heat and cook for 15 minutes until the potatoes are cooked.

Puree the soup in stages in a blender or food processor until smooth. Fill the blender or processor not more than one-third full to prevent burns.

Add the soup back to the pot and heat until it is fully warmed. Serve right away. Serve in separate bowls with toasted fennel seeds on top.

Nutritional Information: Calories: 149 kcal, protein: 6 g, carbohydrates: 28 g, Fat: 1.5 g, Cholesterol: 0.5 mg, Fiber: 3 g

Minestrone soup

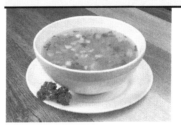

Preparation time: 5 minutes/**Cooking Time:** 35 minutes/**Total time:** 20 minutes

Servings: 4/**Difficulty Level:** Easy

Ingredients:

- 1/2 cup of chopped onion
- 1 tablespoon of olive oil
- 1/3 cup of chopped celery
- 4 cups of low-sodium fat-free chicken broth
- 1 diced carrot,
- 2 large seeded and chopped tomatoes,
- 1 minced garlic clove,
- 1/2 cup of whole-grain uncooked small shell pasta
- 2 tablespoons of chopped fresh basil.
- 1/2 cup of chopped spinach
- 1 small, diced zucchini (about 1 cup)
- 1 can of no-salt-added kidney beans (16 ounces or about 1 1/2 cups) drained.

Instructions

Heat the olive oil in a wide saucepan over medium heat. Add the celery, onion, and carrots. Cook for approximately 5 minutes, or until the vegetables are softened.

Cook for another minute after adding the garlic. Add the beans, tomatoes, broth, spinach, and pasta. Over high heat, bring to a boil. Reduce heat to low and cook for 10 minutes. Toss in the zucchini. Cook for another 5 minutes, covered.

Remove the pan from the heat and add the basil. Immediately ladle into separate bowls and serve.

Nutritional Information: Calories: 200 kcal, protein: 11 g, carbohydrates: 30 g, Fat: 4 g, Cholesterol: 0 mg, Fiber: 7.1 g

Colombian Cream of Avocado Soup

Preparation time: 10 minutes/**Cooking Time:** 0 minutes/**Total time:** 10 minutes

Servings: 8/**Difficulty Level:** Easy

Ingredients:

- 1 cup of light silken tofu (patted dry, drained)
- 3 medium avocados (pitted halved)
- 1/8 teaspoon of black pepper
- 1/2 cup of fat-free milk and 1/4 cup of fat-free milk (as needed) divided or use 1/2 cup of low-sodium fat-free vegetable broth.
- 1/4 teaspoon of salt
- 2 tablespoons of fresh lime juice
- 1/4 cup of fat-free sour cream
- 2 medium limes (cut into 4 wedges)
- 1/4 - 1/2 cup of fresh chopped Cilantro (optional) OR 1/4 - 1/2 cup of chopped fresh chives (optional)

Instructions

Process the tofu, avocados, 1/2 cup of milk, salt, lime juice, and pepper in a food processor or blender until smooth, adding the remaining 1/4 cup of milk if the soup is thicker than desired.

To serve, ladle the soup into bowls. Scoop 1 1/2 teaspoons of sour cream on top of each. Serve with cilantro and lime wedges as garnish. Serve immediately.

Nutritional Information: Calories: 149 kcal, protein: 5 g, carbohydrates: 9 g, Fat: 11.5 g, Cholesterol: 2 mg, Fiber: 7 g

Mexican Chicken Soup

Preparation time: 5 minutes/**Cooking Time:** 30 minutes/**Total time:** 35 minutes

Servings: 6/**Difficulty Level:** Easy

Ingredients:

- 2 tsp. of extra virgin olive oil or canola oil
- 1 14.5- oz. of canned, no-salt-added, kernel corn (drained, rinsed)
- 1 medium chopped bell pepper (green or red),
- 1 15.5- oz. of low-sodium, or no-salt-added, kidney beans (drained, rinsed)
- 2 tsp. of ground cumin
- 1 large chopped onion.
- 1/2 cup of chopped Cilantro
- 1 medium seeded, diced, jalapeño (remove seeds)
- 5 cup of low-sodium fat-free chicken broth
- 2 cloves of garlic (minced) OR 1 tsp. of garlic powder
- 1 large, diced tomato.

- 1.5 lb. skinless, boneless chicken breasts (fat discarded, 1-inch cubes)

Instructions

In a large saucepan, heat the oil over medium heat. Add and cook for 5-7 minutes, often turning until onion, bell pepper, and jalapeño are soft. Cook for another minute after adding the garlic and cumin. Drain, rinse and put aside the beans and corn in a colander.

Increase the heat to high and bring the broth to a quick simmer. Cook until the chicken is no longer pink, approximately 5 minutes. Stir in the beans, tomato, corn, and Cilantro, cover, and cook for 10 minutes over medium heat. Garnish with additional cilantro leaves (if desired) and serve hot.

Nutritional Information:

Calories: 281 kcal, protein: 33 g, carbohydrates: 27 g, Fat: 5 g, Cholesterol: 73 mg, Fiber: 4.3 g

Italian Bean Soup

Preparation time: 10 minutes/**Cooking Time:** 35 minutes/**Total time:** 45 minutes

Servings: 18 servings/**Difficulty Level:** Easy

Ingredients:

- 1 1/2 tablespoons of Italian seasoning
- 15 ounces' great northern beans, canned.
- 30 ounces of canned pinto beans,
- 15 ounces of canned red kidney beans,
- 1 medium chopped onion,
- 15 ounces of canned Italian-style tomatoes,
- 46 ounces of canned tomato juice; low sodium
- 15 ounces of vegetable broth,
- 1/4 teaspoon of black pepper
- 15 ounces of canned green beans,
- 1/4 teaspoon of garlic powder

Instructions

Place beans in a colander once they have been opened. To remove salt, rinse under running water. Allow the water to drain. Fill a large stockpot halfway with water. Remove the onion's brown layers, cut off the ends, and

rinse. Place flat side down after cutting in half lengthwise. Slice the onion into strips while keeping it together. To create dice, turn 1/4 and slice again. Any large pieces should be chopped up. Place into the stockpot. Place green beans in a strainer and rinse under running water to remove sodium. Drain it. Tomato juice, vegetable broth, tomatoes, green beans, pepper, Italian seasoning, and garlic powder should all be added at this point. Cook for 30 minutes by covering it. Serve with whole-wheat rolls or Italian or French bread.

Nutritional Information: Calories: 365 kcal, protein: 22 g, carbohydrates: 68 g, Fat: 2 g, Cholesterol: 0 mg, Fiber: 5.7 g

Lentil Stew

Preparation time: 10 minutes/**Cooking Time:** 1 hour 20 minutes/**Total time:** 1 hour 30 minutes/**Servings:** 8 servings/**Difficulty Level:** Medium

Ingredients:

- 6 cups of water
- 1 tablespoon of margarine
- 15 ounces of low sodium canned tomatoes,
- 1/2 teaspoon of oregano
- 1 onion
- 1/4 teaspoon of garlic powder
- 1-pound lentils
- 8 carrots
- 1 teaspoon of Worcestershire sauce
- 6 celery stalks

Instructions

Remove the onion's ends and peel away the brown layers. To eliminate any dirt, run it underwater. Place the flat side of the onion on the cutting board after cutting it in half lengthwise. Slice across the onion from one side to the other, then turn the slices over and slice across the onion from the widest to the tiniest side. Cut into tiny chunks. Melt the margarine in a large saucepan over medium heat. Add and cook until the onions are soft. Add the lentils, oregano, Worcestershire sauce, water, and garlic powder. Bring to a boil, covered. Reduce the heat to low and cook for 45 minutes. While the lentils are simmering, Carrots should be washed and placed on a chopping board. Lentils should be rinsed.

Both ends should be cut off. Start slicing thin slices from the tiny end. Set it aside. Celery stalks should be washed and placed on a chopping board. Both ends should be cut off, and the lengths should be chopped into shorter lengths. Place these pieces next to each other. Cut longer sections half lengthwise to make them all approximately the same size. Cut across the ends of the pieces until they're all cut up. Put them aside. After 45 minutes, add carrots and celery to lentils. Cover and continue to cook for another 30 minutes, or until the veggies are soft. Toss in the tomatoes. Serve after fully cooked.

Nutritional Information: Calories: 257 kcal, protein: 18 g, carbohydrates: 45 g, Fat: 2 g, Cholesterol: 0 mg, Fiber: 12.8 g

Cream of Celery Soup

Preparation time: 5 minutes/**Cooking Time:** 25 minutes/**Total time:** 30 minutes

Servings: 8 servings/**Difficulty Level:** Medium

Ingredients:

- 3 tablespoons of olive oil, divided.
- 1 bunch of celery (1 1/4 pounds)
- 2 cups of chopped yellow onions.
- 4 finely chopped cloves of garlic,
- 1 tablespoon of chopped fresh thyme.
- ¾ teaspoon of ground fennel seed
- 1 teaspoon of lemon zest
- ½ teaspoon of salt
- 1 ½ tablespoon of fresh tarragon leaves
- 4 cups of chicken broth; no salt added.
- ½ cup of heavy cream
- 2 cups of fresh baby spinach
- ⅛ teaspoon of ground white pepper
- 1 tablespoon of lemon juice

Instructions

Remove the celery leaves (approximately 1/2 cup) and put them aside. To make 4 cups of celery, chop the stalks. (Save any leftover stalks) Heat 1 tablespoon of oil over medium-high heat in a large, heavy saucepan. Cook, often turning, until the celery stalks, thyme, onions, and garlic are cooked, for about 8 to 10 minutes. Cook, stirring periodically, for 30 seconds after adding the lemon zest and ground fennel. Bring the mixture to a boil with the broth and salt. Cook, stirring periodically, for 5 to 6 minutes, or until the celery is tender. Cook for 1 minute, stirring periodically, over medium-high heat with the tarragon, spinach, and lemon juice. Remove the pan from the heat.

Transfer the soup to a blender in batches if necessary. Remove the centerpiece from the blender and secure the lid to enable steam to escape. Cover the opening with a clean cloth. Process on low speed for 45 seconds, gradually increasing to high speed until the mixture is smooth. (Alternatively, use an immersion blender to blend the soup in the pot until smooth, approximately 2 minutes; be careful when blending hot liquids.) Add the cream and white pepper and mix well. Pour the soup into 8 bowls, top with the leftover celery leaves, and drizzle the remaining 2 tablespoons of oil.

Nutritional Information: Calories: 141 kcal, protein: 3.2 g, carbohydrates: 8.4 g, Fat: 10.9 g, Cholesterol: 17 mg, Fiber: 0.7 g

Butternut Squash Soup

Preparation time: 5 minutes/**Cooking Time:** 40 minutes/**Total time:** 45 minutes

Servings: 4 servings/**Difficulty Level:** Medium

Ingredients:

- 1/8 Tsp of Cinnamon
- 3 Cups of No-Sodium Chicken Broth
- 1 Tbsp. of Olive Oil
- 1/8 Tsp of Nutmeg
- 1 Medium Chopped Onion,
- 3 Large peeled and grated Carrots,
- 4 Cups of cubed Butternut Squash

Instructions

In a large pan, heat the olive oil. Cook the onion. Cinnamon and nutmeg will be added at this point. Continue to sauté. Combine the squash, broth, and carrots in a large mixing bowl. Boil until the potatoes are tender. Using an immersion blender, puree the mixture. Makes around 1/12 cup of servings for four people.

Nutritional Information: Calories: 142.9 kcal, protein: 2.4 g, carbohydrates:24.8 g, Fat: 3.7 g, Cholesterol: 0 mg, Fiber: 2 g

Chicken Barley Soup

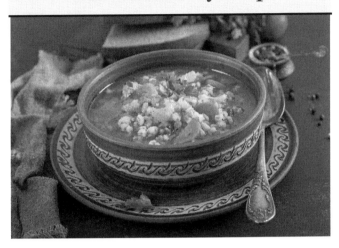

Preparation time: 10 minutes/**Cooking Time:** 1 hour 25 minutes/**Total time:** 1 hour 35 minutes/**Servings:** 5 servings/**Difficulty Level:** Medium

Ingredients:

- 1/2 cup of medium pearl barley
- 1 (2 to 3 pounds) broiler/fryer chicken, cut up
- 1 cup chopped celery.
- 1/2 teaspoon of pepper
- 8 cups of water
- 1-1/2 cups of chopped carrots
- 1 teaspoon of chicken bouillon granules
- 1/2 cup of chopped onion
- 1 teaspoon of salt, optional
- 1/2 teaspoon of rubbed sage.
- 1/2 teaspoon of poultry seasoning
- 1 bay leaf

Instructions

Cook chicken in water in a large stockpot until tender. Remove the fat from the soup once it has cooled. Remove the chicken and set it aside until it is cold enough to handle. Remove the flesh from the bones, toss out the bones, and chop the meat into cubes. Return the meat, along with the other ingredients, to

the pan. Bring the water to a boil. Reduce the heat to low, cover, and cook for 1 hour, or until the veggies and barley are soft. Bay leaf should be discarded.

Nutritional Information: Calories: 259 kcal, protein: 31 g, carbohydrates:22 g, Fat:5 g, Cholesterol: 44 mg, Fiber: 6 g

Black Bean Soup

Preparation time: 10 minutes/**Cooking Time:** 30-40 minutes/**Total time:** 50 minutes

Servings: 9/**Difficulty Level:** Medium

Ingredients:

- 2 chopped celery rib.
- 1 large chopped carrot.
- 2 Tbsp. of garlic pre-minced
- 1 seeded, stemmed, and chopped red bell pepper.
- 4 15oz cans of no salt added black beans.
- 1 10oz can of no salt added diced tomatoes with green peppers; drained.
- 1 large chopped yellow onion
- 2 cups of unsalted chicken broth
- 1 tsp of ground coriander
- ½ tsp of dried oregano
- 1 Tbsp. of ground cumin
- 1 Tbsp. of olive oil
- 1 bay leaf
- Garnish options: shredded cheese, sliced green onion avocado cilantro, sour cream plain or, Greek yogurt.
- 1 tsp of black pepper to taste.

Instructions

Pre-heat a wide pot or soup pot over medium-high heat for a few minutes. When the olive oil is heated, add the celery and onions and simmer for 2 minutes. Then, add the red pepper and carrot, stirring periodically. Cook for another 2 minutes after adding the garlic.

Coriander, diced tomatoes, black beans, bay leaf, vegetable broth, oregano, cumin, and pepper are added. Reduce to low heat and cook for 25 minutes.

Remove bay leaf from the dish. If you want a thicker, creamier soup, use the immersion blender to purée a portion of the soup but don't fully blend it. If you don't have an immersion blender, pour 2 to 3 cups of the soup into a blender and puree until smooth. Return the pureed soup to the pot and stir well. To serve, pour the soup into bowls and top with preferred toppings while still warm.

Nutritional Information: Calories: 89 kcal, protein: 4.1 g, carbohydrates: 14.8 g, Fat: 1.8 g, Cholesterol: 4 mg, Fiber: 10.7 g

African Peanut Stew

Preparation time: 10 minutes/**Cooking Time:** 35 minutes/**Total time:** 45 minutes

Servings: 6/**Difficulty Level:** Medium

Ingredients:

- 2 sweet potatoes, cubed
- 2 tablespoons canola oil
- 1/2 teaspoon minced garlic
- 3 tablespoons fresh ginger, minced
- 2 tablespoons ground coriander
- 1/2 teaspoon cayenne pepper
- 4 cups onion, chopped
- 1 cup tomatoes, chopped
- 1 eggplant, cubed
- 1/2 cup water
- 1 cup zucchini, chopped
- 1 cup green bell pepper, chopped
- 2 cups low sodium tomato juice
- 1/2 cup reduced-fat peanut butter

Instructions

Steam or boil sweet potato cubes until tender. Heat oil in a large skillet over medium-high heat. Sauté garlic, ginger, coriander, and cayenne pepper for 1 minute. Add onions and cook until soft. Add tomatoes, eggplant, and water; simmer for 10 minutes. Add zucchini and bell pepper; continue to simmer for 20 minutes, or until all vegetables are tender. Add sweet potatoes to the stew along with tomato juice and peanut butter. Stir well and simmer on very low heat.

Nutritional Information: Calories: 173 kcal, protein: 4 g, carbohydrates: 31 g, Fat: 5 g, Cholesterol: 0 mg, Fiber: 7 g

Beef Vegetable Soup

Preparation time: 5 minutes/**Cooking Time:** 1 hour 50 minutes/**Total time:** 1 hour 55 minutes/**Servings:** 8/**Difficulty Level:** Medium

Ingredients:

- 1 1/2 pounds round steak, cut in 1h-inch (1.3-cm) pieces
- 1 cup onion, coarsely chopped
- 1/2 cup celery, sliced
- 4 potatoes, cubed
- 4 cups reduced-sodium beef broth
- 1 cup cabbage, coarsely chopped
- 4 cups frozen mixed vegetables, thawed
- 2 cups canned no-salt-added tomatoes

Instructions

Brown meat in a skillet and transfer to slow cooker. Add onion, celery, and potatoes. Pour broth over. Cook on low for 8 to 10 hours. Add cabbage, mixed vegetables, and tomatoes. Turn to high and cook for 30 minutes to 1 hour, or until vegetables are done.

Nutritional Information: Calories: 373 kcal, protein: 37 g, carbohydrates: 48 g, Fat: 4 g, Cholesterol: 49 mg, Fiber: 8 g

Mock Crab Soup

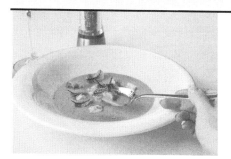

Preparation time: 10 minutes/**Cooking Time:** 20 minutes/**Total time:** 30 minutes

Servings: 4/**Difficulty Level:** Medium

Ingredients:

- 1-pound flounder
- 2 cups low sodium chicken broth
- 2 cups canned no-salt-added tomatoes, diced

- 1/2 cup frozen corn, thawed
- 1/2 cup frozen peas, thawed
- 1 1/2 teaspoons seafood seasoning
- 1/2 teaspoon black pepper
- 1/2 teaspoon cayenne pepper

Instructions

Shred the fish (processing in a food processor with a little broth does this easily). Place all ingredients in a large saucepan and simmer for 10 minutes, or until fish and vegetables are cooked.

Nutritional Information: Calories: 178 kcal, protein: 26 g, carbohydrates: 14 g, Fat: 2 g, Cholesterol: 54 mg, Fiber: 3 g

Beef stew with fennel and shallots

Preparation time: 10 minutes/**Cooking Time:** 1 hour 30 minutes/**Total time:** 1 hour 40 minutes/**Servings:** 6/**Difficulty Level:** Medium

Ingredients:

- 2 tablespoons of canola oil or olive oil
- 1 pound boneless 1 1/2-inch cube of lean beef stew meat, trim off fat
- 3 large, chopped shallots (3 tablespoons)
- 1/2 trimmed and thinly vertically sliced fennel bulb,
- 2 fresh thyme sprigs
- 3/4 teaspoon of ground black pepper, divided.
- 3 tablespoons of plain all-purpose flour
- 3 cups of no-salt vegetable broth or stock
- 1 bay leaf
- 4 large peeled red-skinned or white potatoes, 1-inch chunks.
- 1/2 cup of red wine, optional (not included in the analysis)
- 4 large, peeled carrots, 1-inch chunks
- 18 small boiling onions halved crosswise.
- 1/3 cup of fresh flat-leaf (Italian) parsley finely chopped.
- 3 clean portobello mushrooms, 1-inch chunks

Instructions

On a dish, spread out the flour. By using flour, cover the beef cubes. Heat the oil in a wide, heavy saucepan over medium heat. Add meat, cook, occasionally rotating, until the beef is browned on both sides, approximately for 5 minutes. Remove the meat from the pan with a slotted spoon and put it aside.

Over medium heat, add the shallots and fennel to the pan and cook until softened and gently brown, for about 7 to 8 minutes. Add 1/4 teaspoon of pepper, thyme sprigs, and bay leaf. For 1 minute, sauté it.

Return the meat to the pan and, if using, add the vegetable stock and wine. Bring to a boil, lower to low heat, cover, and cook for 40 to 45 minutes, or until the meat is cooked.

Add potatoes, onions, carrots, and mushrooms. The liquid will not fully cover the veggies, but as the mushrooms soften, more liquid will accumulate. Cook for another 30 minutes, or until the veggies are soft.

Remove the bay leaf and thyme sprigs. Combine the parsley and the remaining 1/2 teaspoon of pepper in a mixing bowl. Serve immediately after ladling into individual warmed bowls.

Nutritional Information: Calories: 244 kcal, protein: 21 g, carbohydrates: 22 g, Fat: 8 g, Cholesterol: 48 mg, Fiber: 4.5 g

White chicken chili

Preparation time: 5 minutes/**Cooking Time:** 25 minutes/**Total time:** 30 minutes

Servings: 8/**Difficulty Level:** Medium

Ingredients:

- 2 cans of (15 ounces each) white beans; low-sodium, drained.
- 1 can (10 ounces) of white chunk chicken
- 4 cups of chicken broth; low-sodium
- 1 can (14.5 ounces) of diced tomatoes; low-sodium
- 1/2 medium chopped green pepper,
- 1 medium chopped onion,
- 2 minced garlic cloves,
- 1 medium chopped red pepper,
- 2 teaspoons of chili powder
- 3 tablespoons of chopped fresh Cilantro.
- 1 teaspoon of dried oregano
- 1 teaspoon of ground cumin
- 8 tablespoons of shredded Monterey Jack cheese; reduced-fat.
- Cayenne pepper, to taste

Instructions

Combine the chicken, tomatoes, beans, and chicken broth in a large soup pot. Simmer, covered, over medium heat.

Spray a nonstick frying pan with cooking spray in the meanwhile. Sauté the peppers, onions, and garlic for 3 to 5 minutes, or until the veggies are tender.

In a soup saucepot, add the onion and pepper mixture. Add the chili powder, oregano, cumin, and cayenne pepper to taste. Cook, occasionally stirring, for approximately 10 minutes, or until all veggies are tender.

Pour into bowls that have been warmed. Serve with 1 tablespoon of cheese and 1 tablespoon of Cilantro.

Nutritional Information: Calories: 212 kcal, protein: 19 g, carbohydrates: 25 g, Fat: 4 g, Cholesterol: 27 mg, Fiber: 4.5 g

Creamy asparagus soup

Preparation time: 5 minutes/**Cooking Time:** 20 minutes/**Total time:** 25 minutes

Servings: 6/**Difficulty Level:** Medium

Ingredients:

- 1/2 pound of fresh asparagus, 1/4-inch pieces
- 2 cups of peeled and diced potatoes
- 2 chopped stalks of celery,
- 1/2 cup of chopped onion
- 2 tablespoons of butter
- 4 cups of water
- Cracked black pepper, to taste.
- 1 1/2 cups of fat-free milk
- 1/2 cup of whole-wheat flour
- Lemon zest, to taste

Instructions

Combine the asparagus, potatoes, asparagus, celery, onions, and water in a large soup pot over high heat. Bring the water to a boil. Reduce the heat to low, cover, and cook for 15 minutes, or until the veggies are soft. Add the butter and mix well. Whisk together the milk and flour in a small bowl. Slowly pour the mixture into the soup pot while continuously stirring. Increase the heat to medium-high and continue to whisk for approximately 5 minutes, or until the soup thickens. Remove the pan from the heat. To taste, add cracked black pepper and lemon zest. Warm bowls are perfect for serving.

Nutritional Information: Calories: 140 kcal, protein: 6 g, carbohydrates: 22 g, Fat: 4 g, Cholesterol: 11 mg, Fiber: 1.8 g

Curried Cream of tomato soup with apples

Preparation time: 10 minutes/**Cooking Time:** 40 minutes/**Total time:** 50 minutes

Servings: 8/**Difficulty Level:** Medium

Ingredients:

- 1 1/2 cups of finely chopped onion.
- 2 tablespoons of olive oil
- 1 cup of finely chopped celery.
- 3 cups of canned tomatoes with no-salt-added, drained.
- 1 teaspoon of minced garlic
- 1/2 teaspoon of thyme
- 1 tablespoon of curry powder, or to taste.
- Ground black pepper, to taste
- 1 bay leaf
- 1 1/2 cups of apple cubes
- 1 cup of long-grain brown rice
- 1 cup of fat-free milk
- 6 cups of low-sodium chicken or vegetable broth

Instructions

Heat the oil in a soup pot over medium heat. Add the chopped celery, onion, and garlic. Cook for approximately 4 minutes, or until the vegetables are soft. Cook for 1 minute while tossing in the curry powder.

Add the bay leaf, tomatoes, black pepper, thyme, and rice to a large mixing bowl. Keep stirring continuously. Pour in the broth. Return to a boil, then reduce to low heat for approximately 30 minutes. Remove the bay leaf when the rice is tender.

Fill a food processor or blender halfway with soup and purée until smooth. Cook until well heated. Return the soup to the pot and stir in the apple cubes and milk. Immediately ladle into individual hot bowls and serve.

Nutritional Information: Calories: 205 kcal, protein: 8 g, carbohydrates: 32 g, Fat: 5 g, Cholesterol: 1 mg, Fiber: 3 g

Creamy Mushroom Soup

Preparation time: 5 minutes/**Cooking Time:** 35 minutes/**Total time:** 40 minutes

Servings: 7/**Difficulty Level:** Medium

Ingredients:

- 4 cups of water
- 1 clove garlic
- 4 tsp of chicken bouillon; no sodium
- 2 Tbsp. of olive oil
- 4 cups of coarsely chopped mushrooms,
- 2 cups of 1% milk
- 1/4 Cup of sherry
- 4 Tbsp. of flour
- 1 medium finely chopped onion,
- Parsley
- 1/2-1 tsp of Italian herbs

Instructions

Heat the oil and then add the onion, mushrooms, and garlic. Cook for 5 minutes with the lid on the pan. Stir occasionally. Stir in the flour and herbs. Bullion should be mixed with hot water and added gently to the pan, stirring constantly. Simmer for 20 minutes. Stir in the sherry. Warm the milk in the pan. Garnish as desired with parsley.

By changing the flour quantity, you may make it thinner or thicker. Use just 2 tablespoons of flour, but it will be too thin to serve as a sauce.

If you need salt, use sea salt, and sprinkle it into your bowl when you're ready to eat; you'll need less.

Nutritional Information: Calories: 92.6 kcal, protein: 3.1 g, carbohydrates: 8.8 g, Fat: 4.4 g, Cholesterol: 1.7 mg, Fiber: 3 g

Autumn Soup

Preparation time: 5 minutes/**Cooking Time:** 25-30 minutes/**Total time:** 35 minutes

Servings: 6/**Difficulty Level:** Medium

Ingredients:

- 1 large peeled and cubed sweet potato,
- 2-1/2 cups of peeled, cubed butternut squash
- 1/4 cup of thawed concentrate orange juice
- 2 tablespoons of minced chives
- 3 medium sliced carrots,
- 1/4 teaspoon of salt
- 3 cups of fat-free milk
- 1 tablespoon of toasted sesame seeds,
- 3 tablespoons of sour cream; reduced-fat.
- 1/4 teaspoon of pepper

Instructions

In a large saucepan, put the sweet potato, squash, and carrots in a steamer basket over 1 inch of water. Bring to a boil, reduce to low heat, and steam for 12-16 minutes, or until the vegetables are soft. Allow cooling slightly. Add the veggies and juice concentrate to the food processor. Process till smooth covered.

Stir in the salt, milk, and pepper in a large pot. Cook and stir over low heat until well heated (do not boil). Serve with 1 teaspoon of chives, 1 1/2 tablespoons of sour cream, and 1/2 teaspoon of sesame seeds on top of each serving.

Nutritional Information: Calories: 166 kcal, protein: 7 g, carbohydrates: 33 g, Fat: 1 g, Cholesterol: 5 mg, Fiber: 5.7 g

Broccoli Soup

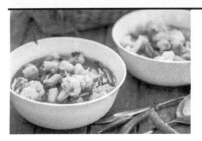

Preparation time: 5 minutes/**Cooking Time:** 25 minutes/**Total time:** 30 minutes

Servings: 4/**Difficulty Level:** Medium

Ingredients:

- 1/4 cup of diced celery
- 1 1/2 cups of chopped broccoli
- 1/4 cup of chopped onion
- 2 cups of nonfat milk
- 1 cup of chicken broth; low-sodium
- 2 tablespoons of cornstarch
- 1 dash of pepper
- 1/4 teaspoon of salt
- 1/4 cup of grated Swiss cheese
- 1 dash of ground thyme

Instructions:

In a saucepan, add the veggies and broth. Bring to a boil, then reduce to low heat and simmer until the veggies are soft, approximately 8 minutes. Combine the pepper, milk, salt, cornstarch, and thyme in a mixing bowl; stir in the cooked veggies.

Cook, stirring continuously, for approximately 5 minutes, or until the soup has gently thickened and the mixture has just started to boil. Remove the pan from the heat. Stir in the cheese until it is completely melted.

Nutritional Information: Calories: 118 kcal, protein: 7 g, carbohydrates: 15.9 g, Fat: 1 g, Cholesterol: 5 mg, Fiber: 3.1 g

Brunswick Stew

Preparation time: 10 minutes/**Cooking Time:** 1 hour 20 minutes/**Total time:** 1 hour 30 minutes/**Servings:** 8/**Difficulty Level:** Medium

Ingredients:

- 15 ounces of low sodium tomato, canned.
- 4 cups of water
- 1 medium chopped onion,
- 2 skinless, boneless chicken breasts
- 15 ounces of butter beans
- 2 teaspoons of vegetable oil
- 15 ounces of corn

Instructions

Boil four cups of water. Cook for 30 minutes, until chicken breasts are cooked through. Allow the chicken to cool in the broth. Cut it into bite-size pieces when the chicken has cooled enough to handle. Using paper towels, spoon, or ice cubes, skim the fat from the chicken stock. Soup can be made using broth. Take 8 cups and measure them. The remainder of the stock can be used for anything else. Remove the brown layers from the onion by cutting the ends off. Cut into small bits using a chef's knife. In a large saucepan, heat the oil until it is very hot. Add and cook until the onions are soft. Add and cook for 30 minutes, or until chicken, butterbeans, tomatoes with their juices, and corn are cooked.

Nutritional Information: Calories: 257 kcal, protein: 25 g, carbohydrates: 34 g, Fat: 4 g, Cholesterol: 36 mg, Fiber: 5 g

Alaskan Cod Chowder

Preparation time: 10 minutes/**Cooking Time:** 35 minutes/**Total time:** 45 minutes
Servings: 6/**Difficulty Level:** Medium

Ingredients:

- 1 cup of diced onion
- 3 tablespoons of extra-virgin olive oil
- ½ cup of all-purpose flour
- 1 cup of diced celery
- ¾ teaspoon of Old Bay seasoning; reduced-sodium.
- 1 tablespoon of Worcestershire sauce
- ¼ teaspoon of salt
- 4 cups of fish or seafood stock; reduced-sodium.
- ¼ teaspoon of ground pepper
- 3 cups of diced red potatoes
- 1 cup of whole milk
- 2 cups of chopped green beans.
- For Garnish, Chopped plum tomatoes.
- 1 pound of Alaskan cod, 1-inch pieces
- For Garnish, Chopped fresh dill.

Instructions

In a wide saucepan over medium heat, heat the oil. Cook, often stirring, until onion and celery are softened and brown; it will take 3 to 6 minutes. Cook, constantly stirring, for 1-minute longer after adding the flour, Old Bay seasoning, salt, Worcestershire sauce, and pepper to the veggies. Bring the milk and fish (or seafood) stock to a moderate boil, stirring continuously.

Add the potatoes and green beans and bring to a low simmer. Simmer, uncovered, for 12 to 15 minutes, or until the potatoes are cooked, stirring occasionally. Cook, often tossing, for 2 to 4 minutes, or until cod is cooked through. If preferred, garnish with dill and tomatoes.

Nutritional Information: Calories: 270 kcal, protein: 18.6 g, carbohydrates: 29.1 g, Fat: 8.9 g, Cholesterol: 33.8 mg, Fiber: 3.2 g

Chapter 11: Chicken Recipes

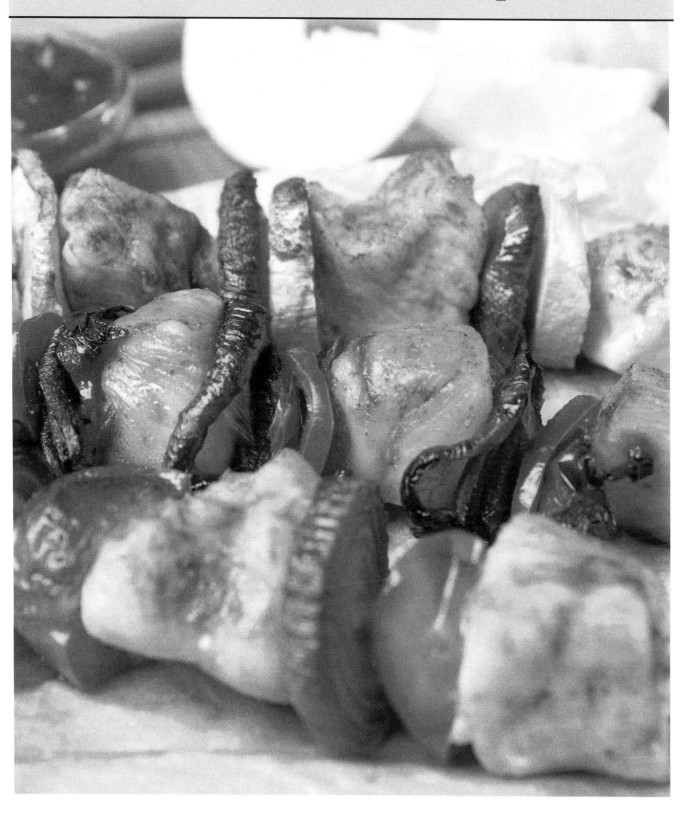

Chicken-Apricot Casserole

Preparation time: 10 minutes/**Cooking Time:** 55 minutes/**Total time:** 1 hour 5 minutes/**Servings:** 4/**Difficulty Level:** Medium

Ingredients:

- 2 chopped garlic cloves,
- 1 sliced onion,
- 2 teaspoons of ground cumin
- 8 chicken thighs,
- 1 1/4 cup of chicken broth; reduced-sodium.
- 2 tsp of ground coriander
- 5 pitted and quartered apricots,
- 2 tbsp of canola oil
- 3 carrots, halved crosswise, 6 to 8 thick fingers,
- Chopped fennel leaves.
- Salt and pepper to taste.

Instructions
Fennel should be split lengthwise and then cut crosswise into slices on a cutting board. In a large pan, heat the oil and cook the chicken thighs, flipping periodically, until golden brown on both sides, for about 5 to 10 minutes. Remove it from the pan. Sauté the garlic and onion in the pan for approximately 5 minutes, or until tender and golden. Add all of the spices and cook for 1 minute before adding the stock.

Return the chicken and the fennel and carrots to the pan. Bring the water to a boil. Stir thoroughly, then cover and cook for 30 minutes, or until the chicken is cooked. Take off the cover. If there is too much liquid, decrease it somewhat by boiling. Stir the apricots into the casserole gently to blend. Cook for another 5 minutes over low heat. Season with salt and pepper to taste. Serve with a sprinkling of fennel leaves.

Nutritional Information: calories: 280 kcal, protein: 26 g, carbohydrates: 18 g, Fat: 13 g, Cholesterol: 49.5 mg, Fiber: 0.7 g

Pasta with grilled chicken, white beans, and mushrooms

Preparation time: 10 minutes/**Cooking Time:** 20 minutes/**Total time:** 30 minutes

Servings: 6/**Difficulty Level:** Medium

Ingredients:

- 1/2 cup of chopped white onion.
- 1 tablespoon of olive oil
- 1 cup of white beans, cooked or canned (no salt added)
- 2 skinless, boneless chicken breasts, 4 ounces each
- 1 cup of sliced mushrooms
- 1/4 cup of chopped fresh basil.
- 2 tablespoons of chopped garlic
- 12 ounces of uncooked roselle pasta
- black pepper: ground, to taste
- 1/4 cup of grated Parmesan cheese

Instructions
In a charcoal grill, create a fire, or heat a broiler or gas grill. Spray the broiler pan or grill rack gently with cooking spray spaced 4 to 6 inches away from the heat source. For 5 minutes, grill or broil each side of the chicken until it turns brown and is cooked through. Allow 5 minutes for the chicken to rest on a chopping board before slicing into strips.

Heat the olive oil in a large nonstick frying pan over medium heat. Sauté the mushrooms and onions for approximately 5 minutes, or until they are soft. Combine the basil, garlic, white beans, and grilled chicken pieces in a large mixing bowl. Keep it warm.

Bring a big saucepan 3/4 full of water to a boil. Add and cook pasta for 10 to 12 minutes, or according to package instructions, until the pasta is al dente (tender). Drain all of the water from the pasta. Add the mixture of chicken to the pasta in the saucepan. Toss to distribute the ingredients properly. Distribute the spaghetti amongst the plates. Garnish with 1 tablespoon of Parmesan cheese and black pepper on top of each. Serve right away.

Nutritional Information: Calories: 341 kcal, protein: 21 g, carbohydrates: 53 g, Fat: 5 g, Cholesterol: 30 mg, Fiber: 4 g

Lemon Rosemary Chicken

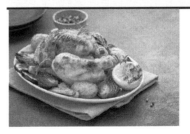

Preparation time: 10 minutes plus marination time/**Cooking Time:** 60 minutes

Total time: 3 hours 10 minutes/**Servings:** 8/**Difficulty Level:** Easy

Ingredients:

- 1 whole chicken, 3 to 4 pounds (1.4 to 1.8 kg)
- 1/2 cup lemon juice
- 1 teaspoon dried rosemary

Instructions

Split chicken in half, cutting along backbone and breastbone. Place in a resalable plastic bag with lemon juice and rosemary. Marinate for at least two hours, turning frequently. Preheat the grill, making one side hot and the other low heat. Cook over the low side with grill covered, turning several times, for about 1 hour or until done. Discard the skin.

Nutritional Information: Calories: 33 kcal, protein: 5 g, carbohydrates: 1 g, Fat: 1 g, Cholesterol: 17 mg, Fiber: 0 g

Chicken Zucchini Pie

Preparation time: 5 minutes /**Cooking Time:** 40 minutes/**Total time:** 45 minutes

Servings: 6/**Difficulty Level:** Medium

Ingredients:

- 1 cup cooked chicken breast, cubed
- 1 cup zucchini, cubed
- 1 cup tomatoes, chopped
- 1 cup onion, chopped
- 1/4 cup Parmesan cheese, shredded
- 1 cup skim milk
- 1/2 cup Reduced-Fat Biscuit Mix
- 1/2 cup egg substitute
- 1/4 teaspoon black pepper

Instructions

Preheat the oven to 400°F (200°C, or gas mark 6) and coat a 9-inch (23-cm) pie plate with nonstick vegetable oil spray. Mix chicken, zucchini, tomatoes, onion, and cheese and spoon evenly into the prepared pie plate. Beat remaining ingredients in a blender or with a wire whisk until smooth. Pour evenly over the chicken mixture. Bake for 35 minutes, or until a knife inserted

in the center comes out clean. Let stand 5 minutes before cutting.

Nutritional Information: Calories: 156 kcal, protein: 15 g, carbohydrates: 15 g, Fat: 4 g, Cholesterol: 25 mg, Fiber: 1 g

Chicken Etouffee

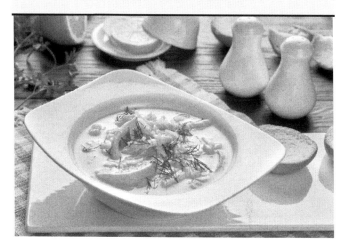

Preparation time: 10 minutes /**Cooking Time:** 25 minutes/**Total time:** 35 minutes

Servings: 4/**Difficulty Level:** Medium

Ingredients:

- 2 tablespoons unsalted margarine
- 1 cup onion, chopped
- 1 tablespoon flour
- 1-pound boneless chicken breasts
- 3/4 cup water
- 2 tablespoons lemon juice
- 2 tablespoons no-salt-added tomato paste
- 1/4 teaspoon cayenne pepper
- 2 tablespoons scallions, sliced
- 1 tablespoon dried parsley

Instructions:

In a saucepan with a tight-fitting lid, melt margarine, add onion, and cook over medium heat until tender. Stir in the flour, blend well. Add chicken, water, lemon, tomato paste, and cayenne pepper. Cook over low heat for 15 minutes, adding more water if necessary. Add scallions and parsley. Serve over steamed rice.

Nutritional Information: Calories: 208 kcal,

protein: 27 g, carbohydrates: 8 g, Fat: 7 g, Cholesterol: 66 mg, Fiber: 1 g

Paella with chicken, leeks, and tarragon

Preparation time: 10 minutes /**Cooking Time:** 1 hour 20 minutes

Total time: 1 hour 30 minutes/**Servings:** 4/**Difficulty Level:** Medium

Ingredients:

- 2 thinly sliced leeks (whites only),
- 1 teaspoon of olive oil; extra-virgin
- 3 minced garlic cloves,
- 1 small, sliced onion,
- 2 chopped large tomatoes,
- 1 pound skinless boneless, chicken breast, strips of 1/2-inch-wide & 2 inches' long
- 2/3 cup of brown rice; long-grain
- 1 sliced red pepper,
- 2 cups of unsalted, fat-free chicken broth
- 1 teaspoon of tarragon, /to taste.
- 1/4 cup of fresh parsley; chopped.
- 1 lemon, slash into 4 wedges
- 1 cup of frozen peas

Instructions:

Heat the olive oil in a large nonstick frying pan over medium heat. Add the garlic, leeks, onions, and chicken strips. Cook for 5 minutes, or until the veggies are transparent and slightly browned the chicken. Continue to sauté for another 5 minutes with the red pepper slices and tomatoes. Add the tarragon, rice, and broth and mix it well. Bring the water to a boil.

Reduce the heat to low, cover, and cook for approximately 10 minutes. Stir in the peas and continue to cook, uncovered, for 45 to 60 minutes, or until the rice is soft and the liquid is absorbed.

To serve, divide the mixture amongst separate dishes. One tablespoon of parsley and one lemon slice is used as a garnish on each plate.

Nutritional Information: Calories: 378 kcal, protein: 35 g, carbohydrates: 46 g, Fat: 6 g, Cholesterol: 82 mg, Fiber: 7 g

Chicken Curry

Preparation time: 10 minutes /**Cooking Time:** 6 hours 25 minutes/**Total time:** 6 hours 35 minutes/**Servings:** 5/**Difficulty Level:** Medium

Ingredients:

- 5 medium potatoes, diced
- 3/4 cup green bell peppers, coarsely chopped
- 3/4 cup onion, coarsely chopped
- 1-pound boneless chicken breasts, cubed
- 2 cups canned no-salt-added tomatoes
- 1 tablespoon ground coriander
- 1 1/2 tablespoons paprika
- 1 tablespoon ground ginger
- 1/4 teaspoon cayenne pepper
- 1/2 teaspoon turmeric
- 1/4 teaspoon cinnamon
- 1/8 teaspoon ground cloves
- 1 cup low sodium chicken broth
- 2 tablespoons cold water
- 1/4 cup cornstarch

Instructions

Place potatoes, green bell peppers, and onion in the slow cooker. Place chicken on top. Mix tomatoes and the next 8 ingredients (through chicken broth). Pour over chicken. Cook on low 8 to 10 hours or high 5 to 6 hours. Remove chicken and vegetables. Turn heat to high. Stir cornstarch into water. Add to cooker. Cook for 15 to 20 minutes, or until sauce is slightly thickened.

Nutritional Information: Calories: 438 kcal, protein: 30 g, carbohydrates: 74 g, Fat: 2 g, Cholesterol: 53 mg, Fiber: 8 g

Honey-Mustard Fruit-Sauced Chicken

Preparation time: 10 minutes /**Cooking Time:** 60 minutes/**Total time:** 1 hour 10 minutes/**Servings:** 6/**Difficulty Level:** Easy

Ingredients:

- 6 boneless chicken breasts
- 1 cup fruit cocktail, in juice
- 2 tablespoons red wine vinegar

- 2 tablespoons honey
- 2 tablespoons honey mustard

Instructions

Preheat oven to 350°F (180°C, or gas mark 4). Place chicken breasts in a roasting pan. Puree fruit cocktail, vinegar, honey, and mustard in a blender. Pour over chicken. Bake for 50 to 60 minutes, or until done.

Nutritional Information: Calories: 122 kcal, protein: 17 g, carbohydrates: 11 g, Fat: 1 g, Cholesterol: 41 mg, Fiber: 1 g

Chili Chicken Breasts

Preparation time: 50 minutes /**Cooking Time:** 25 minutes/**Total time:** 1 hour 15 minutes/**Servings:** 4/**Difficulty Level:** Easy

Ingredients:

- 2 tablespoons olive oil
- 1/3 cup lime juice
- 2 tablespoons chopped green chilis
- 1/4 teaspoon garlic powder
- 4 boneless chicken breasts
- 4 ounces (11 5 g) low-fat Swiss cheese
- Salsa, for serving

Instructions

In a 9-inch (23-cm) square baking pan, stir the olive oil, lime juice, chilis, and garlic powder. Add chicken breasts; marinate in the refrigerator for at least 45 minutes, turning once. Remove chicken from marinade; drain. Grill or sauté chicken for 7 minutes; turn over and continue cooking for 6 to 8 minutes, or until done. Top each chicken breast with a slice of cheese. Continue cooking until cheese begins to melt. Serve with salsa.

Nutritional Information: Calories: 195 kcal, protein: 25 g, carbohydrates: 3 g, Fat: 9 g, Cholesterol: 51 mg, Fiber: 0 g

Rotisserie-Flavored Chicken Breasts

Preparation time: 10 minutes /**Cooking Time:** 45 minutes/**Total time:** 55 minutes

Servings: 4/**Difficulty Level:** Easy

Ingredients:

- 1/4 cup honey
- 1 teaspoon paprika
- 1 teaspoon onion powder
- 1/2 teaspoon black pepper
- 1/2 teaspoon dried thyme
- 1/4 teaspoon garlic powder
- 4 boneless chicken breasts

Instructions

Preheat oven to 325°F (170°C, or gas mark 3). Mix honey, paprika, onion powder, black pepper, thyme, and garlic powder. Rub onto chicken. Roast for 45 minutes, or until done, occasionally basting with pan juices.

Nutritional Information: Calories: 195 kcal, protein: 25 g, carbohydrates: 3 g, Fat: 9 g, Cholesterol: 51 mg, Fiber: 0 g

Chicken tamales

Preparation time: 10 minutes /**Cooking Time:** 1 hour 30 minutes/**Total time:** 1 hour 40 minutes/**Servings:** 4/**Difficulty Level:** Medium

Ingredients:

- 1 tablespoon of canola oil
- 12 corn husks; dried
- 2 skinless, boneless chicken breasts, 12 ounces total (9 ounces is cooked)
- 2 roasted and diced red bell peppers,
- 1 large diced yellow onion,
- 2 diced ribs of celery,
- 4 finely diced cloves of garlic,
- 1 fresh finely diced chili pepper,
- 2 cups of vegetable stock
- 1/2 cup and 2 tablespoons of stone-ground cornmeal (masa)
- 1 tablespoon of ground black pepper
- 1 tablespoon of minced fresh oregano
- 1 tablespoon of cumin seed

Instructions

Soak corn husks for one hour in a bowl of water. Cook the chicken breasts in a large pan over medium heat for 2 minutes on each side, or until it turns golden brown. Take the chicken out of the pan. Sauté the veggies (save the garlic) in the pan for 10 minutes or until gently browned. Add the garlic and cook for another 2 minutes.

Return the chicken to the pan, along with the vegetable stock and seasonings. Reduce the heat to a low simmer. Cook for 20 minutes, or until the chicken reaches an internal temperature of 165 degrees F. Remove the chicken and set it aside to cool.

Add the stone-ground cornmeal to the leftover liquid and cook until the liquid is fully absorbed. Put it aside. Split the chicken. Drain corn husks well and pat dry. Spread the masa mixture on each husk and lay it flat. Distribute the pulled chicken among them. Then add the veggies on top, like a burrito, fold, and roll.

Tamales may be baked at 375°F for 15 minutes or steamed for 30 minutes in a covered colander over the boiling water. Tamales may also be wrapped in nonstick foil and grilled for approximately 5 minutes. Cook until the meat reaches an internal temperature of 165 degrees Fahrenheit. To consume, unwrap the package.

Nutritional Information: Calories: 284 kcal, protein: 26 g, carbohydrates: 27 g, Fat: 8 g, Cholesterol: 54 mg, Fiber: 9.4 g

then add the onion, mushrooms, carrots, and parsley. Cook for about 10 minutes, or until the onions start to brown. Add the walnuts, black pepper, wild rice, and chicken stock. Bring to a boil, then reduce to low heat. Cook for 40 minutes with the cover on.

Meanwhile, heat the remaining oil in a sauté pan. Brown the chicken breasts on both sides, approximately 3 minutes for each side. Cook until the internal temperature reaches 165 degrees Fahrenheit. Remove the chicken from the pan and keep it warm. In a heated pan, add chopped squash and beets. Cook for 15-20 minutes over medium heat, or until squash starts to color and both ingredients are cooked. Toss in the balsamic vinegar, cranberries, chopped greens, and rice mixture to combine and loosen any cooked pieces from the pan's bottom. Serve by dividing the mixture among four bowls and topping with pieces of chicken breasts.

Nutritional Information:

Calories: 413 kcal, protein: 26 g, carbohydrates: 57 g, Fat: 9 g, Cholesterol: 41 mg, Fiber: 9.4 g

Hearty chicken bowl

Preparation time: 10 minutes /**Cooking Time:** 1 hour 30 minutes/**Total time:** 1 hour 40 minutes/**Servings:** 4/**Difficulty Level:** Easy

Ingredients:

- 1 tablespoon of balsamic vinegar
- 2 cups of sliced carrots
- 1 tablespoon of canola oil, divided.
- 2 tablespoons of fresh minced parsley
- 1 cup of diced yellow onion
- 2 tablespoons of chopped walnuts
- 1 cup of fresh mushrooms
- 2 1/2 cups of chicken stock; no-salt-added.
- 1 cup of fancy wild rice; uncooked
- 2 skinless, boneless chicken breasts (4 ounces each)
- 1 tablespoon of black pepper fresh ground
- 2 cups of beet tops; chopped (greens)
- 1 cup of diced red beets
- 2 tablespoons of dried cranberries
- 1 cup of butternut squash; peeled and diced.

Instructions

Heat half of the oil in a saucepan over medium heat,

Boiled Chicken

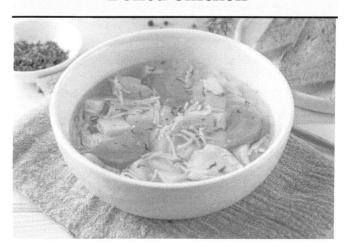

Preparation time: 10 minutes /**Cooking Time:** 1 hour 30 minutes/**Total time:** 1 hour 40 minutes/**Servings:** 8/**Difficulty Level:** Easy

Ingredients:

- 3 unpeeled carrots, smash into chunks
- 1 whole chicken (3 pounds)
- 2 stalks of celery, smash into chunks
- 1 large unpeeled halved onion,
- water to cover.
- 1 tablespoon of whole peppercorns

Instructions

Cover with water in a large saucepan, combine the onion, chicken, celery, carrots, and peppercorns. Then, bring to a boil, lower to low heat, and simmer for 90 minutes until the chicken flesh falls from the bone. Remove the chicken and set it aside to cool before shredding or chopping the flesh

Nutritional Information: Calories: 186 kcal, protein: 16.3 g, carbohydrates: 4.5 g, Fat: 11.1 g, Cholesterol: 46.1 mg, Fiber: 9.4 g

Chicken and Mint Coleslaw Wraps

Preparation time: 10 minutes /**Cooking Time:** 15 minutes/**Total time:** 25 minutes

Servings: 6/**Difficulty Level:** Medium

Ingredients:

- ⅛ teaspoon of salt
- 4 (6-ounce) boneless skinless, chicken breast halves
- □ cup of fresh lemon juice
- Cooking spray
- 2 teaspoons of sugar
- 1 tablespoon of fresh ginger; bottled ground
- 3 cups of angel hair coleslaw
- ¼ teaspoon of red pepper; crushed.
- ½ cup of chopped fresh mint.
- 6 flour tortillas(8-inch)
- 1 poblano chile, seeded, halved lengthwise, and thinly sliced.

Instructions

Using a meat mallet or rolling pin, pound each chicken breast half to 1/4-inch thickness between two sheets of heavy-duty plastic wrap. Season chicken with salt and pepper. Over medium-high heat, place a coated with cooking spray wide nonstick skillet. Add the chicken and cook for 4 1/2 minutes for each side, or until cooked through. Cut the chicken into small strips on a chopping board. Combine the juice, sugar, ginger, and red pepper in a large mixing bowl. Toss in the chicken strips, mint, coleslaw, and chili to coat thoroughly. Toasted tortillas should be warmed according to the package instructions. Distribute the chicken mixture equally among the tortillas and wrap them up. Each rolled tortilla should be cut in half crosswise.

Nutritional Information:

Calories: 304 kcal, protein: 32.6 g, carbohydrates: 31.2 g, Fat: 6.1 g, Cholesterol: 71 mg, Fiber: 3 g

Chicken Pot Pie

Preparation time: 10 minutes /**Cooking Time:** 30 minutes/**Total time:** 40 minutes

Servings: 8/**Difficulty Level:** Easy

Ingredients:

- 2 pounds' boneless chicken breasts
- 2 cups low sodium chicken broth
- 1 cup onion, coarsely chopped
- 1 cup carrot, sliced
- 1 1/3 cups frozen peas, thawed
- 213 cup flour
- 1 cup water
- 1 tablespoon dried parsley
- 1 teaspoon dried thyme
- 6 potatoes, peeled and diced
- 1 cup skim milk

Instructions

Preheat broiler. Place chicken and broth in a slow cooker or Dutch oven and cook until chicken is done. Remove chicken from broth chop coarsely. Strain any fat from broth and add enough water to make 5 cups (1.2 L). Return broth to Dutch oven. Add onions, carrots, and peas and cook for 15 minutes, or until carrots are tender. Add flour to water in a jar with a tight-fitting lid. Shake until dissolved. Add to broth and cook until thickened. Stir in chicken, parsley, and thyme. While the chicken mixture is cooking, boil potatoes until done. Mash with milk. Drop mashed potatoes by spoonful onto the top of the chicken mixture. Broil until potatoes start to brown.

Nutritional Information: Calories: 411 kcal, protein: 36 g, carbohydrates: 61 g, Fat: 2 g, Cholesterol: 66 mg, Fiber: 7 g

Grilled Southwestern Chicken Breasts

Preparation time: 35 minutes /**Cooking Time:** 20 minutes/**Total time:** 55 minutes

Servings: 4/**Difficulty Level:** Easy

Ingredients:

- 4 boneless chicken breasts
- 1/4 cup olive oil
- 2 tablespoons Dijon mustard
- 1 tablespoon rice wine vinegar
- 1 teaspoon black pepper
- dash hot pepper sauce
- 1/4 cup lime juice
- 2 tablespoons cilantro

Instructions

Pound the chicken breasts to 1h-inch (1.3-cm) thickness and place all ingredients in a 1-gallon (3.8-L) resalable plastic bag or a bowl and cover. Marinate in the TIP. Serve with rice and grilled corn. Refrigerator for at least 30 minutes. Grill over medium heat for 20 minutes or until done.

Nutritional Information: Calories: 209 kcal, protein: 17 g, carbohydrates: 2 g, Fat: 15 g, Cholesterol: 41 mg, Fiber: 0 g

Lebanese Chicken and Potatoes

Preparation time: 10 minutes /**Cooking Time:** 60 minutes/**Total time:** 1 hour 15 minutes/**Servings:** 6/**Difficulty Level:** Easy

Ingredients:

- salt to taste
- 8 medium peeled and quartered potatoes,
- 4 crushed cloves of garlic,
- ground white pepper; to taste.
- 1 cup of fresh lemon juice
- 8 chicken pieces; cut up.
- ½ cup of olive oil; extra virgin

Instructions

Preheat the oven to 425 degrees Fahrenheit (220 degrees C). In a large baking dish, combine the potatoes and chicken. Season with white pepper and salt to taste. Combine the olive oil, garlic, and lemon juice in a mixing bowl. Pour over the chicken and potatoes. Wrap foil around the dish and bake for 30 minutes. Remove the foil, raise the heat to 475 degrees F (245 degrees C), cook for 30 minutes or until the chicken and potatoes are browned.

Nutritional Information:

Calories: 586 kcal, protein: 26.7 g, carbohydrates: 53.9 g, Fat: 30.5 g, Cholesterol: 65 mg, Fiber: 5 g

Chicken and asparagus tossed with penne

Preparation time: 5 minutes /**Cooking Time:** 25 minutes/**Total time:** 30 minutes

Servings: 2/**Difficulty Level:** Easy

Ingredients:

- 2 minced cloves of garlic,
- 6 ounces skinless boneless, chicken breasts, 1-inch cubes
- 2 teaspoons of dried basil or oregano
- 1 can (14.5 ounces) no salt added, diced tomatoes, including juice.
- 1 cup of asparagus, 1-inch pieces
- 1 tablespoon of Parmesan cheese
- 1 1/2 cups of whole-grain uncooked penne pasta
- 1-ounce soft crumbled goat cheese (about 1 tablespoon)

Instructions

Bring a large saucepan 3/4 full of water to a boil. Add and cook pasta for 10 to 12 minutes, or according to package instructions, until the pasta is al dente (tender). Drain all of the water from the pasta and set it aside.

Boil 1 inch of water in a saucepan with a steamer basket. Cover and steam for 2 to 3 minutes, or until tender-crisp. Toss in the asparagus.

Using cooking spray, coat a large nonstick frying pan. Sauté the chicken and garlic over medium-high heat.

Cook for 5 to 7 minutes, or until the chicken is golden brown. Simmer for 1-minute longer after adding the tomatoes and their juice, as well as the basil or oregano. Combine the chicken mixture, steamed asparagus, cooked pasta, and goat cheese in a large mixing bowl. Toss lightly to ensure that everything is equally distributed.

Divide the pasta mixture evenly between two dishes to serve. Add 1/2 tablespoon of Parmesan cheese to each dish. Serve right away.

Nutritional Information: Calories: 433 kcal, protein: 34 g, carbohydrates: 54 g, Fat: 9 g, Cholesterol: 75 mg, Fiber: 11 g

Chicken and Dumplings

Preparation time: 10 minutes /**Cooking Time:** 50 minutes/**Total time:** 60 minutes

Servings: 6/**Difficulty Level:** Easy

Ingredients:

For Chicken:

- 1 1/2 cups chicken breast, cooked and cubed
- 3 cups low sodium chicken broth
- 3 cups water
- 1 1/2 cups carrot, sliced
- 6 potatoes, peeled and cubed
- 1 cup onion, chopped

For Dumplings:

- 2 cups flour
- 1 tablespoon baking powder
- 2 tablespoons margarine
- 2/3 cup skim milk

Instructions

To make the chicken: Place chicken, broth, water, carrots, potatoes, and onion in a large pan. Bring to a boil.

To make the dumplings: Stir together the flour and baking powder. Cut in margarine until mixture resembles coarse crumbs. Stir in milk until dough holds together in a ball. Drop dumplings on top of boiling chicken mixture with spoonsful. Reduce heat and simmer uncovered for 10 minutes. Cover and simmer 10 minutes more.

Nutritional Information: Calories: 556 kcal, protein: 26 g, carbohydrates: 100 g, Fat: 7 g, Cholesterol: 30 mg, Fiber: 9 g

Chinese Chicken Meatballs

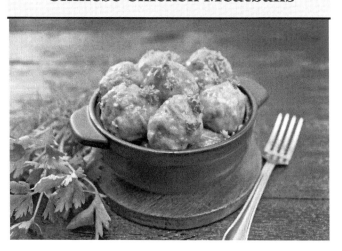

Preparation time: 10 minutes /**Cooking Time:** 40 minutes/**Total time:** 50 minutes

Servings: 4/**Difficulty Level:** Easy

Ingredients:

- 1-pound ground chicken breast
- 1 tablespoon sodium-free beef bouillon
- 1/4 teaspoon ground ginger
- l/s teaspoon garlic powder
- l/s teaspoon black pepper
- 1 tablespoon sherry
- 1/4 cup egg substitute

Instructions

Preheat oven to 350°F (180°C, or gas mark 4). Combine all ingredients. Shape into 1-inch (2.5-cm) balls. Place in a roasting pan that has been well coated with nonstick vegetable oil spray. Roast for 30 to 40 minutes, or until done, turning once.

Nutritional Information: Calories: 153 kcal, protein: 28 g, carbohydrates: 2 g, Fat: 2 g, Cholesterol: 66 mg, Fiber: 0 g

Chicken and Spaghetti Bake

Preparation time: 10 minutes /**Cooking Time:** 35 minutes/**Total time:** 45 minutes

Servings: 6/**Difficulty Level:** Easy

Ingredients:

- 8 ounces spaghetti
- 1/2 cup egg substitute
- 1 cup fat-free cottage cheese
- 1-pound boneless chicken breast, sliced
- 1/2 cup onion, chopped
- 1/2 cup green bell pepper, chopped
- 2 cups canned no-salt-added tomatoes
- 6 ounces no-salt-added tomato paste
- 1 teaspoon sugar
- 1 teaspoon dried oregano
- 1/2 teaspoon garlic powder
- 1/2 cup mozzarella, shredded

Instructions

Preheat oven to 350°F (180°C, or gas mark 4). Cook spaghetti according to package directions. Drain. Mix in egg substitute. Form into a "crust" in a greased 10-inch (25-cm) pie pan. Top with cottage cheese. In a large skillet, cook chicken, onion, and green bell pepper until meat is done and vegetables are tender. Add remaining ingredients except for mozzarella and heat through. Spread over spaghetti and cottage cheese. Bake for 20 minutes. Sprinkle with mozzarella about 5 minutes before the end of baking.

Nutritional Information: Calories: 218 kcal, protein: 27 g, carbohydrates: 22 g, Fat: 2 g, Cholesterol: 46 mg, Fiber: 4 g

Baked chicken and wild rice with onion and tarragon

Preparation time: 30 minutes /**Cooking Time:** 1 hour 25 minutes/**Total time:** 1 hour 55 minutes/**Servings:** 6/**Difficulty Level:** Medium

Ingredients:

- 1 1/2 cups of chopped celery
- 1 pound skinless, boneless, chicken breast halves
- 3/4 cup of uncooked wild rice
- 1 1/2 cups of whole pearl onions

- 2 cups of chicken broth; unsalted
- 1 teaspoon of fresh tarragon
- 1 1/2 cups of dry white wine
- 3/4 cup of long-grain uncooked white rice

Instructions

Preheat the oven to 300 degrees Fahrenheit.

Chicken breasts should be cut into 1-inch chunks. Place the chicken, onions, celery, and tarragon in a nonstick frying pan with 1 cup of unsalted chicken stock. Cook for approximately 10 minutes over medium heat or until the veggies and chicken are cooked. Allow cooling before serving.

Combine the wine, rice, and the remaining 1 cup of chicken stock in a baking dish. Allow 30 minutes to soak. In a baking dish, add the veggies and chicken. Bake for at least 60 minutes after covering it. If the rice becomes too dry, keep an eye on it and add additional liquid as needed. Serve right away.

Nutritional Information: Calories: 313 kcal, protein: 23 g, carbohydrates: 38 g, Fat: 3 g, Cholesterol: 55 mg, Fiber: 4 g

Chicken Gumbo

Preparation time: 10 minutes /**Cooking Time:** 55 minutes/**Total time:** 1 hour 10 minutes/**Servings:** 8/**Difficulty Level:** Medium

Ingredients:

- 2 pounds' boneless chicken breast
- 2 tablespoons minced garlic
- 1/4 cup olive oil
- 1 cup red bell peppers, chopped
- 1 cup onion, chopped
- 1/3 cup flour
- 2 cups canned no-salt-added tomatoes
- 1/2 cup frozen okra, thawed
- 1/4 teaspoon hot pepper sauce
- 1 tablespoon file powder

Instructions

Cook chicken with 5 cups (1.2 L) of water and garlic until tender. Cut chicken into bite-sized pieces. Skim any fat off cooking liquid. Heat the oil in a skillet over medium heat and brown the red bell pepper and onions. Add the flour and brown. Gradually stir in some cooking liquid to make a roux (to desired thickness). Add tomatoes, cover, and simmer for 30 minutes, adding more cooking liquid if needed. Add chicken and okra. Simmer for a few minutes. Season with hot pepper sauce. Add gumbo file powder and stir until blended (lump).

Nutritional Information: Calories: 232 kcal, protein: 28 g, carbohydrates: 11 g, Fat: 8 g, Cholesterol: 66 mg, Fiber: 2 g

Pasta with Chicken and Vegetables

Preparation time: 10 minutes /**Cooking Time:** 30 minutes/**Total time:** 40 minutes
Servings: 6/**Difficulty Level:** Medium

Ingredients:

- 8 ounces' linguine or spaghetti
- 2 tablespoons olive oil
- 1 cup zucchini, cut into strips
- 1/2 cup mushrooms, sliced
- 1/2 teaspoon dried basil
- 1/2 teaspoon minced garlic
- 1 cup skim milk
- 2 cups chicken breast, cooked and cubed
- 1 cup Roma tomatoes, sliced
- 2 tablespoons Parmesan cheese, grated
- 1/8 teaspoon black pepper

Instructions

Cook linguini or spaghetti according to package directions. Meanwhile, heat the oil in a skillet. Add zucchini, mushrooms, basil, and garlic. Cook and stir for 2 to 3 minutes, or until zucchini is crisp-tender. Drain pasta and return to saucepan. Stir in milk, chicken, and zucchini mixture and heat through. Add tomatoes, cheese, and pepper. Toss and serve.

Nutritional Information: Calories: 297 kcal, protein: 23 g, carbohydrates: 31 g, Fat: 9 g, Cholesterol: 74 mg, Fiber: 2 g

Buffalo Chicken Wrap

Preparation time: 15 minutes /**Cooking Time:** 0 minutes/**Total time:** 15 minutes

Servings: 5/**Difficulty Level:** Easy

Ingredients:

- 3 cups leftover cooked, grilled, canned, or rotisserie chicken breast.
- 2 cups chopped romaine lettuce.
- 1 tomato, diced.
- ½ red onion, finely sliced.
- ½ red onion, finely sliced.
- ¼ cup buffalo wing sauce, such as franks Red-hot
- ¼ cup ranch dressing
- Chopped raw cereal (optional)
- 5 small 100 % whole grain low carb wraps

Instructions:

Combine the chicken, lettuce, tomato, onion, wing sauce, dressing, and celery in a large mixing bowl. Place about 1 cup of the mixture onto each wrap. Fold the wrap over the top of the salad, close in the side, and then lightly roll the wrap closed. Use a toothpick to secure the wrap, if needed, and serve.

Nutritional Information: Calories: 200 kcal, protein: 28 g, carbohydrates: 14 g, Fat: 7 g, Cholesterol: 60 mg, Fiber: 8 g

Chicken Nuggets

Preparation time: 10 minutes /**Cooking Time:** 20 minutes/**Total time:** 30 minutes

Servings: 4/**Difficulty Level:** Medium

Ingredients:

- 1/2 cup crushed corn flakes
- 2 tablespoons nonfat dry milk
- 1 tablespoon dried parsley
- 1 tablespoon paprika
- 1 teaspoon onion powder
- 1/4 teaspoon garlic powder
- 1/2 teaspoon poultry seasoning
- 1-pound boneless chicken breasts, cut in strips
- 1/4 cup egg substitute

Instructions

Preheat oven to 350°F (180°C, or gas mark 4). Mix crushed corn flakes and the next 6 ingredients (through poultry seasoning) in a resalable plastic bag. Dip chicken pieces in egg substitute, then place in the bag. Shake to coat evenly. Place on a baking sheet coated with nonstick vegetable oil spray. Bake for 20 minutes, or until chicken is done and coating is crispy.

Nutritional Information: Calories: 167 kcal, protein: 29 g, carbohydrates: 6 g, Fat: 2 g, Cholesterol: 66 mg, Fiber: 1 g

Chicken Veggie Packets

Preparation time: 10 minutes /**Cooking Time:** 20 minutes/**Total time:** 30 minutes

Servings: 4/**Difficulty Level:** Medium

Ingredients:

- 1/2 pound of fresh sliced mushrooms
- 4 skinless, boneless chicken breast halves (4 ounces each)
- 1-1/2 cups of fresh baby carrots
- 1/4 teaspoon of pepper
- 1 cup of pearl onions
- 3 teaspoons of minced fresh thyme
- 1/2 cup of sweet red pepper; julienned
- Lemon wedges, optional
- 1/2 teaspoon of salt, optional

Instructions

Preheat the oven to 375 degrees Fahrenheit. Flatten the chicken breasts to 1/2-inch thickness and put on a heavy-duty foil sheet (12 square). Over the chicken, layer the mushrooms, onions, carrots, and red pepper; season with thyme, pepper, and salt, if preferred. Seal the foil firmly around the chicken and veggies. Place on a baking tray. Cook for approximately 20 minutes, or until the chicken juices flow clear. Serve with lemon wedges if preferred.

Nutritional Information: Calories: 175 kcal, protein: 25 g, carbohydrates: 11 g, Fat: 3 g, Cholesterol: 63 mg, Fiber: 7 g

Avocado, Tomato & Chicken Sandwich

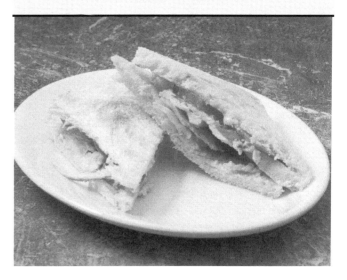

Preparation time: 10 minutes /**Cooking Time:** 15 minutes/**Total time:** 25 minutes

Servings: 1/**Difficulty Level:** Easy

Ingredients:

- ¼ ripe avocado
- 2 slices of multigrain bread
- 2 slices of tomato
- 3 ounces of cooked skinless, boneless chicken breast, sliced.

Instructions

Bread should be toasted. With a fork, mash the avocado and put it over one slice of bread. Add the chicken, tomato, and the second slice of bread on the top. You can poach chicken to use in a recipe if you don't have the cooked chicken. In a skillet or saucepan, place skinless, boneless chicken breasts. Cover with lightly salted water and boil it. Cover, lower heat to a low simmer, and cook until the center is no longer pink, for about 10 to 15 minutes, depending on the size.

Nutritional Information: Calories: 347 kcal, protein: 31.2 g, carbohydrates: 28.4 g, Fat: 12.3 g, Cholesterol: 62.7 mg, Fiber: 7.7 g

Lemony Chicken

Preparation time: 10 minutes plus marination time /**Cooking Time:** 60 minutes

Total time: 1hr. 10 mins/**Servings:** 4/**Difficulty Level:** Easy

Ingredients:

- 1/2 Cup of fresh lemon juice
- 1 1/2 lb. skinned, chicken breast, fat removed.
- 3 tsp of fresh chopped oregano (or 1 tsp dried oregano, crushed)
- 1/2 tsp of paprika
- 2 Tbsp. of white wine vinegar
- 1 medium sliced onion,
- 1/2 Cup of freshly sliced lemon peel,
- black pepper to taste.
- 1/4 tsp of salt

Instructions

Place the chicken in a glass baking dish that measures 13 by 9 by 2 inches. Combine the oregano, lemon juice, lemon peel, vinegar, and onions. Pour it over chicken, cover it, and marinate it overnight in the refrigerator for several hours, flipping occasionally. Season with pepper, salt, and paprika to taste. Cover and bake for 30 minutes at 300°F. Remove the lid and bake it for a further 30 minutes, or until done.

Nutritional Information:

Calories: 179 kcal, protein: 28 g, carbohydrates: 8 g, Fat: 4 g, Cholesterol: 73 mg, Fiber: 0.2 g

Chicken Creole

Preparation time: 5 minutes /**Cooking Time:** 20 minutes/**Total time:** 25 minutes

Servings: 4/**Difficulty Level:** Medium

Ingredients:

- 1 1/2 Cup of chopped (1 large) green pepper,
- 1 Cup of canned tomatoes; low sodium
- 1 1/2 Cup of chopped celery,
- 1 Cup of chili sauce; low-sodium
- 4 media-boned, skinless chicken breast halves, 1-inch strips.

- 1 Tbsp. of fresh basil (or 1 tsp of dried)
- 1/4 Cup of chopped onion,
- 1 Tbsp. of fresh parsley (or 1 tsp of dried)
- 2 minced cloves of garlic,
- 1/4 tsp of crushed red pepper,
- cooking spray; nonstick as needed.
- 1/4 tsp of salt

Instructions

Using nonstick cooking spray, coat a deep skillet. Preheat the pan on high. Cook chicken in a heated skillet for 3–5 minutes, turning occasionally, or until no longer pink. Reduce the temperature. Tomatoes with juice, green pepper, crushed red pepper, low sodium chili sauce, celery, garlic, onion, parsley, basil, and salt are added. Bring to a boil, then turn off the heat. Cover and cook for 10 minutes. Serve with whole wheat pasta or freshly boiled rice.

Nutritional Information: Calories: 274 kcal, protein: 30 g, carbohydrates: 30 g, Fat: 5 g, Cholesterol: 68.4 mg, Fiber: 2.4 g

Chicken Ratatouille

Preparation time: 5 minutes /**Cooking Time:** 25 minutes/**Total time:** 30 minutes

Servings: 4/**Difficulty Level:** Medium

Ingredients:

- 4 medium chicken breast halves, fat removed, skinned, boned, and 1-inch pieces.
- 1 Tbsp. of vegetable oil
- 1 small, peeled eggplant, 1-inch cubes
- 2 unpeeled, thinly sliced zucchini, about 7 inches long,
- 1 medium thinly sliced onion,
- 1/2 lb. fresh sliced mushrooms,
- 1 1/2 tsp of crushed dried basil,
- 1 green medium pepper, 1-inch pieces
- 1 Tbsp. of fresh minced parsley,
- 1 can (16 oz.) of whole tomatoes, cut up.
- Black pepper to taste.
- 1 minced clove of garlic,

Instructions

In a large nonstick skillet, heat the oil. Add the chicken

and cook for 3 minutes, or until it is gently browned. Add eggplant, zucchini, green pepper, onion, and mushrooms. Cook, stirring periodically, for approximately 15 minutes. Toss in the parsley, garlic, tomatoes, basil, and salt & pepper to taste. Cook, occasionally stirring, for approximately 5 minutes, or until the chicken is cooked.

Nutritional Information: Calories: 266 kcal, protein: 30 g, carbohydrates: 21 g, Fat: 8 g, Cholesterol: 66 mg, Fiber: 6.3 g

Caribbean Chicken Stir-Fry

Preparation time: 5 minutes /**Cooking Time:** 25 minutes/**Total time:** 25 minutes

Servings: 4/**Difficulty Level:** Medium

Ingredients:

- 1 can of mixed tropical fruit; coarsely chopped (15 ounces), drained.
- 2 teaspoons of Caribbean jerk seasoning
- 2 teaspoons of cornstarch
- 1/4 cup of water
- 2 packages of brown rice; ready-to-serve (8.8 ounces each)
- 1-pound skinless, boneless chicken breasts, 1/2-inch strips

Instructions

Combine cornstarch and water in a small bowl until smooth. Coat the large skillet with cooking spray. Add the chicken and season with jerk spice. Stir-fry for 3 to 5 minutes, or until the chicken is no longer pink. Add the cornstarch mixture and stir well. Toss in some fruit. Bring to a boil, then reduce to low heat and simmer, constantly stirring, for 1-2 minutes, or until the sauce has thickened. In the meanwhile, cook the rice according to the package instructions. Serve alongside chicken.

Nutritional Information: Calories: 433 kcal, protein: 28 g, carbohydrates: 60 g, Fat: 5 g, Cholesterol: 63 mg, Fiber: 3 g

Grilled Basil Chicken and Tomatoes

Preparation time: 10 minutes plus marination time/**Cooking Time:** 15 minutes

Total time: 25 minutes/**Servings:** 4/**Difficulty Level:** Medium

Ingredients:

- 2 tablespoons of olive oil
- 1/4 cup of fresh basil leaves; tightly packed
- 3/4 cup of balsamic vinegar
- 1/2 teaspoon of salt
- 1 minced garlic clove,
- 4 skinless, boneless chicken breast halves (4 ounces each)
- 8 plum tomatoes

Instructions

In a blender, combine the first five ingredients for the marinade. Four tomatoes are added to a blender; cover and mix until smooth. To grill the remaining tomatoes, cut them in half.

Combine the 2/3 cup of marinade and chicken in a bowl; refrigerate for 1 hour, flipping periodically. Save the rest of the marinade for serving.

Drain the chicken and toss out the marinade. Place the chicken on a grill rack that has been greased over medium heat. Cover and grill chicken for 4-6 minutes on each side, or until a thermometer reads 165°F. Cover and grill tomatoes for 2-4 minutes on each side over medium heat, until gently browned. Serve the chicken and tomatoes with the marinade that was saved.

Nutritional Information:

Calories: 177 kcal, protein: 24 g, carbohydrates: 6.3 g, Fat: 5 g, Cholesterol: 63 mg, Fiber: 0 g

Spinach and Mushroom Smothered Chicken

Preparation time: 10 minutes /**Cooking Time:** 20 minutes/**Total time:** 30 minutes

Servings: 4/**Difficulty Level:** Medium

Ingredients:

- 3 sliced green onions,
- 1-1/2 teaspoons of olive oil
- 3 cups of fresh baby spinach
- 1-3/4 cups of sliced fresh mushrooms
- 4 skinless, boneless chicken breast halves (4 ounces each)
- 2 tablespoons of chopped pecans
- 2 slices of provolone cheese; reduced-fat, halved.
- 1/2 teaspoon of rotisserie chicken seasoning

Instructions

Preheat the grill or the broiler. Heat the oil in a large pan over medium-high heat and cook the green onions and mushrooms until tender. Stir in the pecans and spinach until they are completely wilted. Remove from the heat and set aside to keep warm.

Season the chicken with spices. Grill for 4-5 minutes on each side on an oiled grill rack, covered over medium heat, or broil it on a greased broiler pan keeping 4 inches away from heat until a thermometer registers 165°. Top with cheese and grill or broil until melted. To serve, spoon the mushroom mixture over the top.

Nutritional Information: Calories: 203 kcal, protein: 27 g, carbohydrates: 3 g, Fat: 9 g, Cholesterol: 68 mg, Fiber: 1.5 g

Grilled Chicken Wings

Preparation time: 10 minutes /**Cooking Time:** 25 minutes/**Total time:** 35 minutes

Servings: 8/**Difficulty Level:** Easy

Ingredients:

- 1 ½ pound frozen chicken wings
- Freshly ground black pepper
- 1 teaspoon garlic powder
- 1 cup low salt buffalo wing sauce
- 1 teaspoon extra virgin olive oil

Instructions:

Preheat the grill to 350 degrees F. Season the wings with black pepper and garlic powder. Grill the wings for 15 minutes on each side until they are browned and crispy. Toss the wings with sauce and olive oil and serve warm.

Nutritional Information: Calories: 82 kcal, protein: 7 g, carbohydrates: 1 g, Fat: 6 g, Cholesterol: 27 mg, Fiber: 0 g

Egg roll

Preparation time: 10 minutes /**Cooking Time:** 20 minutes/**Total time:** 30 minutes

Servings: 6/**Difficulty Level:** Easy

Ingredients:

- 2 teaspoons of sesame oil, divided.
- 1 teaspoon minced garlic
- 1 onion finely diced.
- 1-pound extra-lean ground chicken
- 1 ½ tablespoon low-sodium soy sauce
- ½ cup low sodium chicken broth
- 2 teaspoons ground ginger
- ½ teaspoon freshly ground black pepper.
- 4 cups green cabbage chopped or shredded into 1-inch ribbons.
- 1 ½ cups shredded carrots.
- 1 cup fresh bean sprouts
- 2 scallions were finely chopped.

Instructions:

Place a large skillet over medium-high heat. Add 1 teaspoon of sesame oil and garlic. Stir for 1 minute. Add the onion and cook until tender, 1 to 2 minutes. Add the ground chicken. Cook until browned, breaking up the meat into smaller pieces for 7 to 9 minutes. While the meat is browning, mix the remaining 1 teaspoon of the sesame oil, soy sauce, broth, ginger, and black pepper in a small bowl. When the chicken is cooked, stir the sauce into the skillet. Add the cabbage, carrots, and bean sprouts. Stir to combine. Cover the skillet and simmer until the cabbage is tender for 5 to 7 minutes. Serve in a bowl and garnish with the scallions and additional soy sauce to taste.

Nutritional Information:

Calories: 133 kcal, protein: 19 g, carbohydrates: 7 g,

Fat: 3 g, Cholesterol: 14.2 mg, Fiber: 2 g

Jerk Chicken with Mango salsa

Preparation time: 10 minutes plus refrigeration time/**Cooking Time:** 40 minutes

Total time: 60 minutes/**Servings:** 4/**Difficulty Level:** Medium

Ingredients:

- 2 tablespoons extra virgin olive oil
- Juice of 1 lime
- 1 tablespoon minced garlic
- 1 teaspoon ground ginger
- ½ teaspoon dried thyme
- ½ teaspoon cinnamon
- ½ teaspoon ground all spices.
- ½ teaspoon ground nutmeg
- ¼ teaspoon of cayenne pepper
- 1 teaspoon of finely ground black pepper.
- ¼ teaspoon of ground cloves
- 4 boneless, skinless chicken breasts about 1 pound
- 1 cup mango salsa

Instructions:

In a gallon-sized zip-top freezer bag, put the olive oil, lime juice, garlic, ginger thyme, cinnamon, allspice, nutmeg, cayenne, cloves, and black pepper. Tightly seal the bag and gently mix the marinade. Add the chicken breasts to the marinade. Tightly seal the bag and shake to coat the chicken in the marinade. Refrigerate for at least 30 minutes or overnight. Preheat the grill to medium-high heat. Place the chicken on the grill and discard the marinade. Cook the chicken for about 6 minutes on each side or until the breasts are no longer pink in the middle and reach an internal temperature of 165 degrees F or bake the chicken for 25 minutes in preheated oven at 400 degrees F. Let the chicken rest for 5 minutes before slicing. Top the chicken slices with the mango salsa.

Nutritional Information: Calories: 206 kcal, protein: 25 g, carbohydrates: 11 g, Fat: 9 g, Cholesterol: 20.6 mg, Fiber: 1 g

Chicken with Asparagus

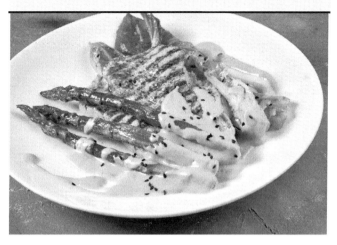

Preparation time: 10 minutes /**Cooking Time:** 40 minutes/**Total time:** 50 minutes

Servings: 4/**Difficulty Level:** Medium

Ingredients:

- 4 boneless chicken breasts
- 1 tablespoon cilantro, chopped
- 2 tablespoons olive oil
- 1/2-pound asparagus, cut in 3-inch (7.5-cm) lengths
- 1 1/2 cups low sodium chicken broth
- 1 tablespoon cornstarch
- 1 tablespoon lemon juice
- 1/2 teaspoon black pepper

Instructions:

Slice the chicken breasts into strips about 1J4-inch (62-mm) thick. Sprinkle with cilantro and toss to coat. Heat the oil in a large frying pan and fry the chicken quickly in small batches, 1 to 2 minutes per side. Remove from pan when no longer pink. Add asparagus and chicken broth to the pan and bring to a boil. Cook for 4 to 5 minutes, or until asparagus is tender. Mix the cornstarch with a little water and stir into the broth. Cook until thickened. Add the chicken. Stir in the lemon juice and pepper. Cook until chicken is heated through.

Nutritional Information: Calories: 170 kcal, protein: 18 g, carbohydrates: 3 g, Fat: 9 g, Cholesterol: 44 mg, Fiber: 0 g

Sweet-and-Sour Chicken

Preparation time: 10 minutes /**Cooking Time:** 35 minutes/**Total time:** 45 minutes

Servings: 4/**Difficulty Level:** Medium

Ingredients:

- 8 1/2 ounces' pineapple chunks, undrained
- 1/2 cup duck sauce, divided
- 2 tablespoons brown sugar
- 1/4 cup rice vinegar
- 1/4 cup orange juice
- 1-pound boneless chicken breasts, cut in l/2-inch (1 .3-cm) pieces
- 1 teaspoon Reduced-Sodium Soy Sauce
- 1-pound frozen oriental vegetable mix, thawed
- 1/4 teaspoon ground ginger
- 2 teaspoons cornstarch
- 1 tablespoon water

Instructions:

Mix juice from pineapple with 1/4 cup (60 ml) duck sauce, brown sugar, vinegar, soy sauce, and orange juice. Set aside. In a large skillet with a tight-fitting lid, add chicken and sauté for 5 minutes, or until no longer pink on the outside. Add soy sauce, pineapple chunks, vegetables, and ginger. Cover and simmer until chicken is done and vegetables are crisp-tender. Stir together water and cornstarch. Add to pan with remaining 1/4 cup (60 ml) duck sauce. Cook until the mixture is thickened and bubbly. Serve over rice.

Nutritional Information:

Calories: 330 kcal, protein: 30 g, carbohydrates: 54 g, Fat: 2 g, Cholesterol: 66 mg, Fiber: 6 g

Chicken and Snow Peas

Preparation time: 10 minutes /**Cooking Time:** 30 minutes/**Total time:** 40 minutes

Servings: 4/**Difficulty Level:** Medium

Ingredients:

- 2 tablespoons olive oil, divided
- 1-pound boneless chicken breasts, sliced
- 1/4 cup egg substitute
- 1/3 cup cornstarch
- 1 1/2 cups onions, sliced
- 1/2 cup green bell pepper, sliced
- 6 ounces snow peas
- 1/4 cup honey
- 2 tablespoons almonds, slivered

Instructions:

Heat 1 tablespoon (15 ml) of the oil in a wok. Dip half the chicken in the egg substitute and dust with cornstarch. Stir-fry for 4 to 5 minutes, or until just cooked. Remove cooked chicken from pan and repeat with remaining chicken. Remove chicken from pan; add the rest of the oil to the wok. Stir fry the onion until it begins to soften. Add the green bell pepper and snow peas and stir-fry for 4 minutes, or until crisp-tender. Add the honey and toss the vegetables in it until well coated. Add the chicken and toss until coated and heated through. Sprinkle the almonds over the top.

Nutritional Information:

Calories: 375 kcal, protein: 31 g, carbohydrates: 38 g, Fat: 11 g, Cholesterol: 66 mg, Fiber: 3 g

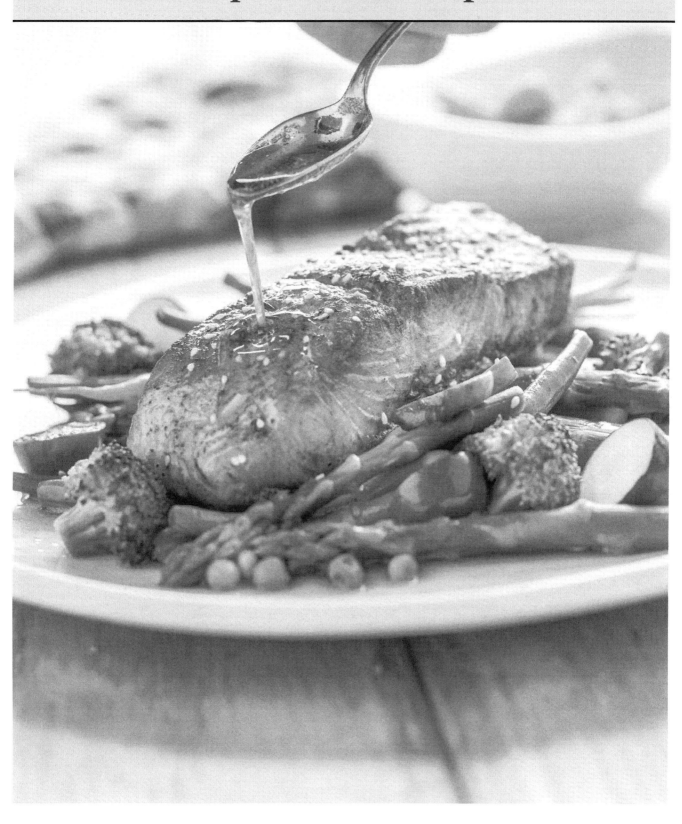

Fish Veracruz

Preparation time: 20 minutes/**Cooking Time:** 30 minutes/**Total time:** 50 minutes

Servings: 8/**Difficulty Level:** Easy

Ingredients

- 1/2 tablespoon of canola oil
- 1/4 cup of lime juice
- 1 small peeled and sliced onion,
- 1/4 cup of seeded and sliced.
- 1 small seeded green bell pepper, strips
- 2 cups of pico de gallo or fresh salsa
- jalapeno pepper,
- 1/2 cup of tomato sauce; no salt added.
- 2 pounds of whitefish fillets, such as sole, tilapia, pollock cod, or halibut
- 1 tablespoon of capers
- 1/2 cup of sliced ripe olives
- 1 lime, 8 wedges
- 4 tablespoons of chopped fresh cilantro, / 4 teaspoons of dried cilantro.

Instructions

In a baking pan of 9-by-13-inch, arrange the fish. Lime juice is sprinkled on top. Refrigerate it for 20 minutes after covering.

Preheat the oven to 425 degrees Fahrenheit. In a large non-stick skillet, heat the oil over medium-high heat. Add the bell pepper, onion, and jalapeño pepper. Cook for 2 minutes, stirring periodically, or until veggies are cooked yet crisp.

Add salsa, olives, tomato sauce, and capers. Bring it to a boil. Reduce heat to low and cook for 1 minute.

Pour sauce over the fish and bake for 20 minutes in a preheated oven or until the fish flakes easily with a fork. With a slotted spatula, remove the fish and veggies from the pan. Serve with lime wedges and cilantro.

Nutritional Information:

Calories: 172 kcal, protein: 23 g, carbohydrates: 11 g, Fat: 4 g, Cholesterol: 57 mg, Fiber: 2.1 g

Provençal Baked Fish with Roasted Potatoes & Mushrooms

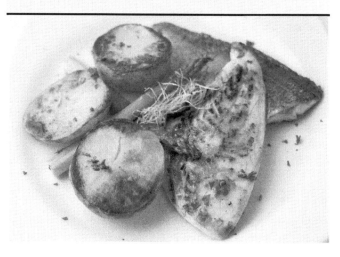

Preparation time: 5 minutes/**Cooking Time:** 55 minutes/**Total time:** 60 minutes

Servings: 4/**Difficulty Level:** Medium

Ingredients:

- 1-pound mushrooms; trimmed and sliced (oyster, shiitake, cremini, or fresh mushrooms),
- 1 teaspoon of herbs de Provence
- 1-pound cubed Gold /red potatoes,
- ¼ teaspoon of salt
- 2 tablespoons of olive oil; extra-virgin, divided.
- ¼ teaspoon of ground pepper
- 14 ounces' grouper, halibut, or cod fillet; 4 portions
- 2 peeled and sliced cloves of garlic,
- Fresh thyme; for garnish
- 4 tablespoons of lemon juice

Instructions

Preheat the oven to 425 degrees Fahrenheit. In a large mixing bowl, combine potatoes, salt, 1 tablespoon oil, mushrooms, and pepper. Fill a baking dish of 9x13-inch halfway with the mixture. Roast for 30 to 40 minutes or until the veggies are barely tender.

Stir in the veggies, followed by the garlic. Arrange the fish on top. Drizzle with the remaining 1 tbsp of oil and lemon juice. Herbes de Provence should be sprinkled on top. Bake for 10 to 15 minutes, or until the salmon is opaque in the middle and flakes readily. If desired, garnish with thyme.

Nutritional Information: Calories: 276 kcal, protein: 24.4 g, carbohydrates: 25.3 g, Fat: 8.8 g, Cholesterol: 48.6 mg, Fiber: 2.8 g

Tuna Couscous

Preparation time: 15 minutes/**Cooking Time:** 10 minutes/**Total time:** 25 minutes

Servings: 4/**Difficulty Level:** Medium

Ingredients

- 1 cup dry couscous
- 2 tablespoons olive oil
- 2 large carrots, thinly sliced
- 4 cups green beans, cut into 1-inch pieces
- 2 yellow zucchinis, sliced in half lengthwise and cut into half rounds
- Sea salt for seasoning
- Freshly ground black pepper for seasoning
- 2 (4-ounce) can chunk albacore tuna

Instructions

Prepare the couscous according to package directions and set aside. In a large skillet, heat the olive oil over medium-high heat. Sauté the carrots until tender-crisp, about 5 minutes. Add the green beans, zucchini, and sauté until the vegetables are tender about 5 minutes. Season the vegetables with salt and pepper. Spoon the couscous into 4 bowls and evenly divide the vegetables between them. Serve topped with tuna.

Nutritional Information: Calories: 357 kcal, protein: 21 g, carbohydrates: 48 g, Fat: 10 g, Cholesterol: 25 mg, Fiber: 8 g

Mediterranean Baked Fish

Preparation time: 5 minutes/**Cooking Time:** 45 minutes/**Total time:** 50 minutes

Servings: 4/**Difficulty Level:** Easy

Ingredients

- 1 large, sliced onion,
- 2 tsp of olive oil

- 1/2 Cup of tomato juice (saved from canned tomatoes)
- 1 can of whole tomatoes, coarsely chopped drained (reserve juice), (16 oz)
- 1 bay leaf
- 1 cup of dry white wine
- 1 lb. fish fillets (flounder, sole, or sea perch)
- 1 minced clove of garlic,
- 1/4 Cup of lemon juice
- 1/2 tsp of crushed dried oregano,
- 1/4 Cup of orange juice
- 1 Tbsp. of freshly grated orange peel,
- 1 tsp of crushed fennel seeds,
- 1/2 tsp of crushed dried thyme,
- black pepper to taste.
- 1/2 tsp of crushed dried basil,

Instructions

In a large non-stick skillet, heat the oil. Add the onion and cook for 5 minutes over medium heat or until tender. Except for the fish, add the other ingredients. Stir thoroughly and cook for 30 minutes, uncovered. Arrange the fish in a baking dish that measures 10 by 6 inches. Cover with a layer of sauce. Bake for 15 minutes at 375°F, uncovered, or until fish readily flakes.

Nutritional Information: Calories: 178 kcal, protein: 22 g, carbohydrates: 12 g, Fat: 4 g, Cholesterol: 56 mg, Fiber: 2.5 g

Baked Swordfish with Vegetables

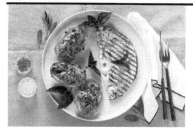

Preparation time: 5 minutes/**Cooking Time:** 55 minutes/**Total time:** 60 minutes

Servings: 4/**Difficulty Level:** Easy

Ingredients

- 4 ounces' mushrooms, sliced
- 1 cup onion, sliced
- 2 tablespoons green bell pepper, chopped
- 2 tablespoons lemon juice

- 1/4 teaspoon dried dill
- 1-pound swordfish steaks
- 4 small bay leaves
- 2 tomatoes, sliced

Instructions

Preheat oven to 400°F (200°C, or gas mark 6). Combine mushrooms, onions, green bell pepper, lemon juice, and dill in a bowl. Line a shallow baking pan with foil. Spread vegetable mixture in the bottom, then arrange swordfish steaks on top. Place a bay leaf on each swordfish steak. Place 2 tomato slices on each swordfish steak. Cover pan with foil and bake for 45 to 55 minutes or until fish flakes easily with a fork.

Nutritional Information: Calories: 165 kcal, protein: 24 g, carbohydrates: 6 g, Fat: 5 g, Cholesterol: 44 mg, Fiber: 1 g

Salmon Skewers

Preparation time: 35 minutes/**Cooking Time:** 30 minutes/**Total time:** 1 hour 10 minutes/**Servings:** 2/**Difficulty Level:** Easy

Ingredients

- ☐ cup of lemon juice
- 2 skinless salmon fillets (6 ounces), 1-inch thick, 2-inch-long strips
- 1 tablespoon of fresh dill; chopped.
- ¼ cup of white wine
- 1 tablespoon of fresh mint; chopped.
- 1 pinch of red pepper flakes; crushed.
- 2 tablespoons of fresh parsley; chopped.
- ¼ cup of olive oil
- 2 tablespoons of minced garlic

Instructions

Preheat the grill to medium-low. In the base of a baking dish, place the salmon. Combine the mint, wine, lemon juice, dill, garlic, parsley, and red pepper flakes in a mixing bowl. Slowly pour in olive oil while stirring thoroughly. Over the fish, pour the mixture. Refrigerate the salmon for no more than 30 minutes after marinating. Thread the fish lengthwise onto metal or moist wooden skewers. Cook until the center is opaque, approximately 4 minutes on each side, over a hot grill. Serve right away.

Nutritional Information: Calories: 561 kcal, protein: 30 g, carbohydrates: 7.8 g, Fat: 43.2 g, Cholesterol: 82.7 mg, Fiber: 1.8 g

Fish Ceviche

Preparation time: 20 minutes/**Cooking Time:** 10 minutes/**Total time:** 30 minutes

Servings: 2/**Difficulty Level:** Medium

Ingredients:

- 1 cucumber
- ½ small red onion
- 1 small mango
- 2 lbs. haddock/ codfish
- 1 tbsp. of sea salt
- 9 limes
- 1½ tbsp. of pink peppercorn
- ½ bunch of cilantro
- 1 small slice of watermelon
- 2 serrano peppers

Instructions

Cut fish into approximately 1/2-inch-long pieces and blanch it for 3 minutes in boiling water and take it out and cool it on ice. Put the fish in a bowl. Add the juice of 5 limes. Allow 10 minutes to marinate in the refrigerator. Meanwhile, combine the pink peppercorn, sea salt, coarsely chopped serrano pepper, cilantro, and cucumber in a mortar and pestle. One lime should be squeezed, and everything should be ground until it resembles an Italian pesto (or use a food processor or blender).

Put the remaining diced cucumber (with skin on) and cubed mango in a dish. Squeeze the remaining limes and add red onion and finely chopped cilantro. Toss together all of the ingredients. Add avocado and marinated fish (and watermelon if using). Mix everything with care. For 5 minutes in the refrigerator, chill it before serving.

Nutritional Information: Calories: 82 kcal, protein: 15 g, carbohydrates: 2.6 g, Fat: 1.3 g, Cholesterol: 37 mg, Fiber: 0.5 g

Classic Blackened Scallops

Preparation time: 10 minutes/**Cooking Time:** 3 minutes/**Total time:** 15 minutes

Servings: 4/**Difficulty Level:** Easy

Ingredients

- 2 tablespoons hot smoked paprika
- 2 teaspoons onion powder
- 1 teaspoon garlic powder
- 1 teaspoon sea salt
- 1 teaspoon of dried thyme
- 1-pound sea scallops, cleaned
- ½ teaspoon of black pepper; freshly ground
- 2 tablespoons olive oil

Instructions

Combine the paprika, onion powder, garlic powder, salt, thyme, and pepper in a small bowl. Pat the scallops dry with a paper towel and dredge them on the top and bottom in the spice mixture. In a wide skillet, heat the olive oil over medium-high heat. Add the scallops to the skillet, ensuring they do not touch each other. Sear on both sides, turning once, for a total of about 3 minutes.

Nutritional Information: Calories: 178 kcal, protein: 20 g, carbohydrates: 6 g, Fat: 8 g, Cholesterol: 37 mg, Fiber: 2 g

Grilled Tuna with Honey-Mustard Marinade

Preparation time: 30 minutes/**Cooking Time:** 20 minutes/**Total time:** 50 minutes

Servings: 4/**Difficulty Level:** Medium

Ingredients

- 1/3 cup red wine vinegar
- 1 tablespoon spicy brown mustard
- 1 tablespoon honey
- 3 tablespoons extra-virgin olive oil
- 1-pound tuna steaks

Instructions

Combine the vinegar, mustard, honey, and olive oil in a jar or covered container; shake to mix well. Put tuna in a resalable plastic bag; add the mustard mixture. Seal the bag and let it marinate for about 20 minutes. Heat the grill. Remove the tuna from the marinade and pour the marinade into a small saucepan. Bring marinade to a boil; remove from heat and set aside. Grill the tuna over high heat for about 2 minutes on each side or to desired doneness. Drizzle with the hot marinade.

Nutritional Information: Calories: 275 kcal, protein: 27 g, carbohydrates: 5 g, Fat: 16 g, Cholesterol: 43 mg, Fiber: 0 g

Herbed Fish

Preparation time: 10 minutes/**Cooking Time:** 30 minutes/**Total time:** 40 minutes

Servings: 4/**Difficulty Level:** Easy

Ingredients

- 2 pounds' perch, or another firm white fish
- 1 tablespoon olive oil
- 1/2 teaspoon garlic powder
- 1/2 teaspoon dried marjoram
- 1/2 teaspoon dried thyme
- 1/8 teaspoon white pepper
- 2 bay leaves
- 1/2 cup onion, chopped
- 1/2 cup white wine

Instructions

Preheat oven to 350°F (180°C, or gas mark 4). Wash fish, pat dry, and place in a 9 x 13-inch (23 x 33-cm) dish. Combine oil with garlic powder, marjoram, thyme, and white pepper. Drizzle over fish. Top with bay leaves and onion. Pour wine over all. Bake, uncovered, for 20 to 30 minutes, or until fish flakes easily with a fork.

Nutritional Information: Calories: 277 kcal, protein: 43 g, carbohydrates: 3 g, Fat: 7 g, Cholesterol: 95 mg, Fiber: 0 g

Cod with Green Bean Curry

Preparation time: 20 minutes/**Cooking Time:** 60 minutes/**Total time:** 1 hour 20 minutes/**Servings:** 4/**Difficulty Level:** Medium

Ingredients

For First Bake:

- ½ pound of trimmed green beans, bite-sized pieces
- 4 plum sliced tomatoes, (Roma)
- 2 minced cloves of garlic,
- 1 sliced white onion,
- salt and ground black pepper to taste.
- 1 tablespoon olive oil, or more as needed.

Curry Mixture:

- 2 teaspoons of curry powder
- 1 ½ cod fillets (6 ounces)
- 2 teaspoons of ground ginger
- 2 tablespoons of water,

Instructions

Preheat an oven to 400 degrees Fahrenheit (200 degrees C). Combine onion, green beans, tomatoes, and garlic in a large glass baking dish. Season it with pepper and salt and toss it with olive oil to coat it.

Bake it, turning periodically, until the onion edges are slightly browned, and the green beans begin to appear dry for approximately 40 minutes in a preheated oven. Meanwhile, combine the curry powder, water, and ginger.

Remove the casserole from the oven and stir veggies, followed by the curry mixture. Increase the oven's temperature to 450 degrees Fahrenheit (230 degrees C). Coat the bottom of the dish with veggies and place the fish on top. Bake for another 25 to 30 minutes, depending on thickness, until the fish is opaque.

Nutritional Information: Calories: 130 kcal, protein: 43 g, carbohydrates: 10.8 g, Fat: 4.2 g, Cholesterol: 23.4 mg, Fiber: 3.6 g

Mediterranean Baked Fish

Preparation time: 5 minutes/**Cooking Time:** 50 minutes/**Total time:** 55 minutes

Servings: 4/**Difficulty Level:** Easy

Ingredients

- 1 large, sliced onion,
- 2 tsp of olive oil
- 1/2 Cup of tomato juice (saved from canned tomatoes)
- 1 can of whole tomatoes, coarsely chopped drained (reserve juice), (16 oz)
- 1 bay leaf
- 1 cup of dry white wine
- 1 lb. fish fillets (flounder, sole, or sea perch)
- 1 minced clove of garlic,
- 1/4 Cup of lemon juice
- 1/2 tsp of crushed dried oregano,
- 1/4 Cup of orange juice
- 1 Tbsp of freshly grated orange peel,
- 1 tsp of crushed fennel seeds,
- 1/2 tsp of crushed dried thyme,
- black pepper to taste.
- 1/2 tsp of crushed dried basil,

Instructions

In a large non-stick skillet, heat the oil. Add the onion and cook for 5 minutes over medium heat or until tender. Except for the fish, add the other ingredients. Stir thoroughly and cook for 30 minutes, uncovered. Arrange the fish in a baking dish that measures 10 by 6 inches. Cover with a layer of sauce. Bake for 15 minutes at 375°F, uncovered, or until fish readily flakes.

Nutritional Information: Calories: 178 kcal, protein: 22 g, carbohydrates: 12 g, Fat: 4 g, Cholesterol: 56 mg, Fiber: 1.5 g

Tuna Fish Tacos

Preparation time: 10 minutes/**Cooking Time:** 10-15 minutes7**Total time:** 25 minutes

Servings: 12/**Difficulty Level:** Easy

Ingredients

- 2 minced cloves garlic,
- 1 tablespoon of olive oil
- 2 teaspoons of ground cumin
- 4 sliced green onions,
- 1 teaspoon of dried oregano
- 4 cans of solid white tuna packed in water: drained (6 ounces)
- 3 dashes of hot sauce
- 4 diced Roma tomatoes,
- 1 pinch of red pepper flakes (optional)
- 12 corn tortillas
- salt and black pepper; ground, to taste

Instructions

In a skillet, heat the olive oil over medium heat. Sauté cumin, green onions, tomatoes, garlic, oregano for 5 minutes, or until tomatoes are very soft. Reduce the heat to a low setting. Mix in the drained tuna, carefully breaking it up into bite-sized pieces. Season it with salt and pepper, as well as red pepper flakes. Cover and simmer for another 2 to 3 minutes, or until tuna has warmed through.

On a microwave-safe dish, stack 6 tortillas and cover with a wet paper towel. Microwave for 15 to 20 seconds, or until malleable. Continue with the remaining tortillas. Overheated tortillas, spoon tuna mixture, and serve it.

Nutritional Information: Calories: 140 kcal, protein: 16.2 g, carbohydrates: 13.2 g, Fat: 2.5 g, Cholesterol: 16.8 mg, Fiber: 1.5 g

Baked Sea Bass and Vegetables

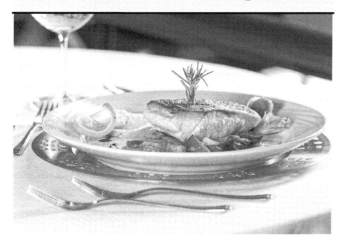

Preparation time: 10 minutes/**Cooking Time:** 40 minutes/**Total time:** 50 minutes

Servings: 4/**Difficulty Level:** Medium

Ingredients

- 4 small, sliced eggplants,
- 1 tablespoon of dried oregano
- 2 tablespoons of olive oil
- 1 tablespoon of dried basil
- salt and black pepper; ground, to taste
- 5 diced Roma tomatoes,
- 1 sliced Roma tomato,

- 4 fillets of sea bass (3 ounces)

Instructions

Preheat an oven to 400 degrees Fahrenheit (200 degrees C). Line a baking dish with aluminum foil, allowing it to hang over the edges.

Combine the oregano, olive oil, salt, basil, and pepper in a large mixing bowl. Next, stir in the eggplant and chopped tomatoes to completely coat them in the oil mixture.

Place the sea bass in the middle of the baking dish and stack veggies on each side of the fish, finishing with sliced tomatoes. Next, raise and fold the edges of the aluminum foil to allow the fish to bake in the vegetable liquid.

Bake them for 35 to 40 minutes in a preheated oven until fish easily flakes with the fork and eggplant is soft.

Nutritional Information: Calories: 359 kcal, protein: 21.3 g, carbohydrates: 29.5 g, Fat: 19.8 g, Cholesterol: 35.1 mg, Fiber: 1.8 g

Fish Wine Chowder

Preparation time: 5 minutes/**Cooking Time:** 40 minutes/**Total time:** 45 minutes
Servings: 8/**Difficulty Level:** Medium

Ingredients

- 1-pound salmon
- 1-pound perch
- 4 slices low sodium bacon
- 1/2 cup onion, chopped
- 1/2 cup celery, chopped
- 1/4 teaspoon minced garlic
- 1 1/2 cups white wine
- 1 1/2 cups water
- 2 potatoes, cubed
- 1/4 teaspoon thyme
- 1 teaspoon parsley
- 3 tablespoons flour
- 3 tablespoons water
- 1/2 cup skim milk

Instructions

Cut fish into cubes; set aside. Cook bacon in a Dutch oven; crumble and set aside. Drain grease from pan. Sauté onion, celery, and garlic until tender. Add wine, water, potatoes, thyme, and parsley. Simmer for 20 minutes, or until potatoes are almost done. Add the fish, cover, and simmer for 10 minutes more. Mix flour and water to form a paste. Stir into soup and simmer until thickened. Stir in milk and reserved bacon.

Nutritional Information: Calories: 306 kcal, protein: 26 g, carbohydrates: 21 g, Fat:9 g, Cholesterol: 62 mg, Fiber: 2 g

Poached Salmon

Preparation time: 5 minutes/**Cooking Time:** 25 minutes/**Total time:** 30 minutes

Servings: 2/**Difficulty Level:** Medium

Ingredients

- 4 cups water
- 2 tablespoons lemon juice
- 1/4 cup carrot, thinly sliced
- 1/2 cup onion, thinly sliced
- 1 bay leaf
- 1 tablespoon fresh dill, chopped
- 1/2-pound salmon fillets

Instructions

Preheat oven to 350°F (180°C, or gas mark 4). Combine all ingredients except salmon in a saucepan and heat to boiling. Reduce heat and simmer for 5 minutes. Place salmon in a glass baking dish large enough to hold salmon in a single layer; pour poaching liquid over. Cover and bake for 20 minutes, or until salmon flakes easily.

Nutritional Information: Calories: 238 kcal, protein: 24 g, carbohydrates: 7 g, Fat: 12 g, Cholesterol: 67 mg, Fiber: 1 g

Halibut with basil tomato salsa

Preparation time: 10 minutes/**Cooking Time:** 15 minutes/**Total time:** 25 minutes

Servings: 4/**Difficulty Level:** Medium

Ingredients

- 1 teaspoon of chopped fresh oregano,
- 2 diced tomatoes (about 1 1/2 cups)
- 1 tablespoon of minced garlic
- 2 tablespoons of fresh basil, chopped.
- 4 halibut fillets, 4 ounces each
- 2 teaspoons of olive oil; extra-virgin

Instructions

Preheat an oven to 350 degrees Fahrenheit. Spray a baking pan of 9-by-13-inch lightly with cooking spray. Combine the basil, oregano, tomato, and garlic in a small bowl. Mix with olive oil.

In a baking pan, arrange the halibut fillets. Spread the tomato sauce on top of the fish. Place it in the oven and bake for 10 to 15 minutes, or until the fish is translucent throughout when checked with the tip of a knife. Immediately transfer to separate plates and serve.

Nutritional Information: Calories: 55 kcal, protein: 22 g, carbohydrates: 4 g, Fat: 4 g, Cholesterol: 55 mg, Fiber: 1 g

Mango Shrimp Kebabs

Preparation time: 10 minutes/**Cooking Time:** 10 minutes/**Total time:** 25 minutes

Servings: 4/**Difficulty Level:** Medium

Ingredients:

- ½ teaspoon of salt
- 2 limes; cut into wedges.
- 1 ½ pound large shrimp; peeled and deveined
- 2 large red bell peppers; 1-inch pieces
- ⅛ teaspoon of black pepper; freshly ground.
- 2 peeled mangoes; 1-inch cubes
- Cooking spray
- 1 small red onion; 1-inch pieces

Instructions

Heat the grill to medium-high heat. Season the shrimp with pepper and salt to taste. Using 8 (12-inch) skewers, alternately thread mango, bell pepper, shrimp, and onion pieces. Grill for 2 minutes on each side, or until shrimp are done, on a grill rack sprayed with cooking spray. Lime wedges should be squeezed over the kebabs.

Nutritional Information: Calories: 277 kcal, protein: 35.8 g, carbohydrates: 27.1 g, Fat: 3.3 g, Cholesterol: 60 mg, Fiber: 4.2 g

Tuna Steaks

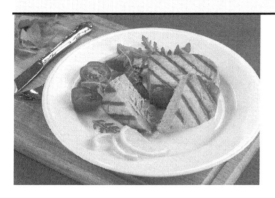

Preparation time: 30 minutes/**Cooking Time:** 10 minutes/**Total time:** 40 minutes

Servings: 2/**Difficulty Level:** Medium

Ingredients

- 2 tablespoons olive oil
- 2 tablespoons lemon juice
- 6 ounces' tuna steaks
- 1/2 teaspoon freshly ground black pepper

Instructions

Combine the olive oil and lemon juice. Marinate the steaks in the mixture for at least 30 minutes, turning occasionally. Heat a skillet over high heat. Add the steaks and cook for 2 minutes. Sprinkle with pepper, turn over, and cook 2 minutes longer.

Nutritional Information: Calories: 247 kcal, protein: 20 g, carbohydrates: 2 g, Fat: 18 g, Cholesterol: 32 mg, Fiber: 0 g

Sun-dried Tomato Pesto Snapper

Preparation time: 5 minutes/**Cooking Time:** 15 minutes/**Total time:** 20 minutes

Servings: 4/**Difficulty Level:** Medium

Ingredients

- 1 sweet onion, cut into ¼-inch slices
- 4 (5-ounce) snapper fillets
- Freshly ground black pepper for seasoning
- ¼ cup sun-dried tomato pesto
- 2 tablespoons finely chopped fresh basil

Instructions

Preheat the oven to 400°F. Line a baking dish with parchment paper and arrange the onion slices on the bottom. Pat the snapper fillets dry with a paper towel and season them lightly with pepper. Place the fillets on the onions and spread 1 tablespoon of pesto on each fillet. Bake until the fish flakes easily with a fork, 12 to 15 minutes. Serve topped with basil.

Nutritional Information: Calories: 199 kcal, protein: 36 g, carbohydrates: 3 g, Fat: 3 g, Cholesterol: 66 mg, Fiber: 1 g

Salmon Patties

Preparation time: 10 minutes/**Cooking Time:** 15 minutes/**Total time:** 35 minutes

Servings: 8/**Difficulty Level:** Medium

Ingredients

- 1 finely diced onion,
- 2 cans of pink salmon (15 ounces)
- 1 cup of cornmeal
- 1 egg, beaten.
- Salt and pepper; to taste.
- 8 crushed saltine crackers,
- 0.15 cup of canola oil
- 1 stalk of celery

Instructions

Combine the egg, salmon, onion, pepper, crackers, salt, and celery in a medium mixing bowl. Mix thoroughly.

Make patties from the salmon mixture and coat them with cornmeal. Warm oil for frying in a wide frying pan over medium-high heat. Place the salmon patties in the oil and cook until golden brown on both sides. Drain thoroughly. Warm the dish before serving.

Nutritional Information: Calories: 237 kcal,

protein: 19.8 g, carbohydrates: 12.3 g, Fat: 11.8 g, Cholesterol: 70.7 mg, Fiber: 1.8 g

Barbequed Steelhead Trout

Preparation time: 5 minutes/**Cooking Time:** 15 minutes/**Total time:** 20 minutes

Servings: 6/**Difficulty Level:** Medium

Ingredients

- ¼ cup of butter, melted.
- 2 pounds of steelhead trout fillets
- ¼ teaspoon of paprika
- 2 tablespoons of lemon juice
- ¼ cup of barbeque sauce
- ⅛ teaspoon of cayenne pepper

Instructions

Preheat the outdoor grill to medium heat and brush the grate liberally with oil. Arrange the fillets of fish on a big sheet of aluminum foil. Brush the fillets with a mixture of butter, paprika, lemon juice, and cayenne pepper. Cook on a hot grill for approximately 10 minutes, or until the fish easily flakes with a fork; coat the fillets with the barbeque sauce and cook for another 2 minutes.

Nutritional Information: Calories: 285 kcal, protein: 28.8 g, carbohydrates: 4.3 g, Fat: 16.2 g, Cholesterol: 100.7 mg, Fiber: 0.1 g

Mussels in Curried Coconut Milk

Preparation time: 5 minutes/**Cooking Time:** 15 minutes/**Total time:** 20 minutes

Servings: 4/**Difficulty Level:** Medium

Ingredients

- 2 tablespoons olive oil
- ½ sweet onion, finely chopped
- 1 tablespoon minced garlic
- 2 teaspoons grated fresh ginger
- 1 tablespoon curry powder
- 1 cup coconut milk
- 1½ pounds fresh mussels, scrubbed and debearded
- 2 tablespoons finely chopped cilantro

Instructions

Heat the olive oil over medium-high heat in a large skillet and sauté the onion, garlic, and ginger until softened for about 3 minutes. Add the curry powder and toss to combine. Stir in the coconut milk and bring to a boil. Add the mussels, cover, and steam until the shells are open, about 8 minutes. Remove any unopened shells and take the skillet off the heat. Stir in the cilantro and serve.

Nutritional Information: Calories: 263 kcal, protein: 9 g, carbohydrates: 9 g, Fat: 23 g, Cholesterol: 16 mg, Fiber: 2 g

Paprika Tilapia

Preparation time: 7 minutes/**Cooking Time:** 10 minutes/**Total time:** 20 minutes

Servings: 2/**Difficulty Level:** Easy

Ingredients

- 2 tilapia fillets
- 1 teaspoon ground paprika
- ½ teaspoon chili powder
- 2 tablespoons avocado oil

Instructions

Sprinkle the tilapia fillets with ground paprika and chili powder. Then heat avocado oil in the skillet for 2 minutes. Put the fish fillets in the hot oil and cook for 3 minutes per side.

Nutritional Information: Calories: 170 kcal, protein: 21.4 g, carbohydrates: 1.7 g, Fat: 3.1 g, Cholesterol: 55 mg, Fiber: 1.2 g

Creole-Style Catfish

Preparation time: 5 minutes/**Cooking Time:** 30 minutes/**Total time:** 35 minutes

Servings: 6/**Difficulty Level:** Medium

Ingredients

- 1 tablespoon olive oil

- 1 cup onion, chopped
- 1/2 cup celery, chopped
- 1/2 cup green bell pepper, chopped
- 1 clove garlic, minced
- 2 cups canned no-salt-added tomatoes
- 1 lemon, sliced
- 1 tablespoon Worcestershire sauce
- 1 tablespoon paprika
- 1 bay leaf
- 1/4 teaspoon dried thyme
- 1/4 teaspoon hot pepper sauce
- 2 pounds' catfish fillets

Instructions

Heat the oil in a large skillet over medium heat. Add the onion, celery, green pepper, and garlic. Cook until soft. Add tomatoes and their liquid. Break the tomatoes with a spoon. Add lemon slices, Worcestershire sauce, paprika, bay leaf, thyme, and hot pepper sauce. Cook, occasionally stirring, for 15 minutes, or until the sauce is slightly thickened. Press fish pieces down into sauce and spoon some of the sauce over the top of the fish. Cover the pan and simmer gently for 10 minutes, or until the fish flakes easily with a fork. Serve over hot cooked rice.

Nutritional Information: Calories: 260 kcal, protein: 25 g, carbohydrates: 9 g, Fat: 14 g, Cholesterol: 71 mg, Fiber: 2 g

Roasted Orange-Fennel Striped Bass

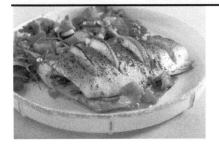

Preparation time: 10 minutes/**Cooking Time:** 35 minutes/**Total time:** 45 minutes

Servings: 4/**Difficulty Level:** Medium

Ingredients:

- 2 tablespoons of olive oil; extra-virgin, divided.
- 1 large fennel bulb (with stalks)
- ¾ teaspoon of kosher salt, divided.
- 6 minced garlic cloves,
- 3 tablespoons of fresh lemon juice
- 2 (1 3/4-pound) cleaned whole striped bass
- ¼ teaspoon of black pepper; freshly ground.
- 1 orange; 8 slices
- Cooking spray

Instructions

Preheat the oven to 400 degrees Fahrenheit. Remove the fronds from the fennel bulb and coarsely chop them to make 1 tablespoon of fronds. Stalks should be removed and discarded. Fennel bulbs are thinly sliced. Over medium-high heat, heat the large nonstick skillet. Swirl in 1 tablespoon of oil to coat it. Add the garlic and sliced fennel to the pan and cook, often turning, for 6 minutes or until gently browned. Add 1/4 teaspoon of salt. Remove the pan from heat and set it aside to cool for 5 minutes.

Make three diagonal incisions in the skin of each fish. Whisk together the remaining 1 tablespoon of oil and the lemon juice. Half of the lemon juice mixture should be rubbed into each fish's flesh, and the other half should be drizzled outside each fish. Sprinkle the remaining 1/2 teaspoon of salt and pepper evenly within the flesh. Place each fish on a jelly-roll pan lined with parchment paper sprayed with cooking spray. Fill each fish with half of the fennel mixture and four orange slices.

Allow resting for 5 minutes after roasting at 400° for 30 mins /until fish flakes readily when checked with a fork. Fennel fronds, if used, should be sprinkled over the fish.

Nutritional Information: Calories: 271 kcal, protein: 33 g, carbohydrates: 11 g, Fat: 10.5 g, Cholesterol: 70 mg, Fiber: 3 g

Thai-Style Fish

Preparation time: 5 minutes/**Cooking Time:** 15-20 minutes/**Total time:** 25 minutes

Servings: 8/**Difficulty Level:** Medium

Ingredients:

- 2 pounds' catfish fillets, cut in 2-inch (5-cm) pieces

- 1/4 cup lime juice
- 1/4 teaspoon red pepper flakes
- 1 tablespoon sesame oil
- 1 cup onion, thinly sliced
- 1 cup celery, sliced
- 1 cup bok choy, shredded
- 1 teaspoon ground ginger
- 1 teaspoon minced garlic
- 1 tablespoon curry powder
- 8 cups low sodium chicken broth
- 2 cups cooked rice

Instructions

Mix catfish, lime juice, and red pepper flakes; set aside. Heat sesame oil in a large saucepan or Dutch oven. Sauté onion, celery, bok choy, ginger, and garlic for 1 minute. Sprinkle with curry powder. Reduce heat and sauté until the onion is soft. Add chicken broth and bring to a boil. Stir in catfish mixture and simmer for 3 minutes, or until catfish is done. To serve, place rice in the center of soup bowls and ladle soup over.

Nutritional Information: Calories: 275 kcal, protein: 24 g, carbohydrates: 18 g, Fat: 12 g, Cholesterol: 53 mg, Fiber: 1 g

Lemon-Pepper Salmon Burgers

Preparation time: 15 minutes/**Cooking Time:** 20 minutes/**Total time:** 35 minutes

Servings: 4/**Difficulty Level:** Medium

Ingredients:

- 2 tsp. of Dijon mustard
- 4 (2.5 oz.) pouches of lemon-pepper salmon
- 1 tsp. Of olive oil mayonnaise
- ½ cup of panko, and 1 tbsp. of panko (gluten-free panko)
- 1 egg
- 1 tsp. Of dried dill weed.
- Juice & zest of ½ lemon
- Dash of cayenne pepper
- Olive oil; for sautéing
- Salt & ground black pepper; to taste.

Instructions:

In a medium mixing bowl, combine all ingredients

until thoroughly mixed (except 1 tablespoon of panko and olive oil for sautéing). Form the mixture into four equal-sized salmon patties and put them on a parchment-lined dish. Refrigerate it for at least 15 mins after topping the patties with half of the leftover panko (1/2 tbsp.), covering them with foil.

In a sauté pan, heat the olive oil over medium heat. Place panko-side down salmon burger patties in the pan. Spread the remaining 1/2 tbsp. Panko equally over the patties. Patties should be cooked for approximately 4-5 mins on each side or until golden.

Nutritional Information: Calories: 403 kcal, protein: 20 g, carbohydrates: 10 g, Fat: 32 g, Cholesterol: 75 mg, Fiber: 3 g

Greek Roasted Fish with Vegetables

Preparation time: 35 minutes/**Cooking Time:** 20 minutes7**Total time:** 55 minutes

Servings: 4/**Difficulty Level:** Medium

Ingredients:

- 2 tablespoons of olive oil
- 1 pound lengthwise halved fingerling potatoes,
- ½ teaspoon of sea salt
- 5 coarsely chopped garlic cloves,
- ½ teaspoon of black pepper; freshly ground.
- 2 medium yellow, red, and orange sweet peppers; cut into rings.
- 4 5 to 6-ounce skinless salmon fillets; fresh or frozen
- 2 cups of cherry tomatoes
- ¼ cup of pitted halved Kalamata olives,
- 1 ½ cups of chopped fresh parsley; (1 bunch)
- 1 lemon
- ¼ cup of fresh finely snipped oregano / 1 Tbsp. of dried crushed oregano,

Instructions

Preheat the oven to 425 degrees Fahrenheit. In a large mixing bowl, place the potatoes. Toss with garlic, 1 tbsp. Of oil, and 1/8 tsp. of salt & black pepper; toss to coat. Cover with foil and transfer to a 15x10-inch baking pan. For 30 minutes, roast it.

In the meanwhile, defrost any frozen fish. Sweet peppers, oregano, parsley, tomatoes, olives, and 1/8 teaspoon of salt & black pepper all go into the same bowl. Drizzle the remaining 1 tbsp. Of oil over the top and toss to coat.

Rinse the fish and pat it dry. Sprinkle fish with remaining 1/4 teaspoon of salt & black pepper to taste. Top potatoes with the sweet pepper mixture and fish. Roast for another 10 minutes, uncovered, or until fish flakes easily. Lemon zest should be removed. Lemon juice should be squeezed over the fish and veggies. Add a dash of zest.

Nutritional Information: Calories: 422 kcal, protein: 32.9 g, carbohydrates: 31.5 g, Fat: 18.6 g, Cholesterol: 78 mg, Fiber: 5.7 g

Steamed Fish with Sesame and Ginger

Preparation time: 10 minutes/**Cooking Time:** 10 minutes/**Total time:** 20 minutes

Servings: 4/**Difficulty Level:** Medium

Ingredients:

Fish

- 3 minced cloves of garlic,
- 2 tbsp of grated fresh ginger
- 1/4 cup of chopped cilantro
- 1/2 tsp of grated lime zest
- 4 tilapia or cod fillets, about 150 g (5 oz) each
- 2 1/2 tsp of dark sesame oil
- Salt to taste

Sauce

- ½ cup of water

- 2 tbsp. of fresh lime juice
- 1/4 cup of cilantro
- 1 tsp of cornstarch that is blended with 1 tbsp. of water.

Instructions

Combine the garlic, lime zest, ginger, and cilantro in a small bowl. Sprinkle the cilantro mixture and salt over the skinned side of the fillets and place them on the work surface. Fillets should be folded in half. Place the folded fish on a heatproof plate and drizzle with sesame oil.

In a pan wide enough to accommodate a plate of fish, place the cake rack and pour water slightly below the cake rack. Bring to a low simmer after covering it.

Place the fish plate on the rack over the boiling water with care. Cover and steam for 5 minutes, or until well done. Transfer the fish to a dish with a slotted spatula and cover loosely to keep it warm.

Pour the cooking juices from the steaming plate into a small saucepan to create the sauce. Add water and lime juice, boil it. Stir in the cornstarch mixture and simmer, constantly stirring, for 1 minute, or until the sauce has gently thickened. Add the cilantro and mix well. Pour the sauce and pass it to a small serving dish to the table.

Nutritional Information:

Calories: 170 kcal, protein: 27 g, carbohydrates: 3 g, Fat: 5 g, Cholesterol: 1 mg, Fiber: 1 g

Stuffed Peppers with Cod

Preparation time: 10 minutes/**Cooking Time:** 25 minutes/**Total time:** 35 minutes

Servings: 4/**Difficulty Level:** Medium

Ingredients:

- 1 minced onion,
- 10 oz. minced cod fillet,
- 4 trimmed, seeded bell peppers,
- 1 teaspoon of ground black pepper
- 1 teaspoon of olive oil
- ¼ cup of coconut cream

Instructions

Combine the onion, cod, and black pepper in a mixing bowl. Then, place the peppers filled with the cod mixture in the saucepan. Add coconut cream and olive oil. Put the cover. Cook the dish for 25 minutes over medium heat.

Nutritional Information: Calories: 152 kcal, protein: 14.6 g, carbohydrates: 12.7 g, Fat: 5.7 g, Cholesterol: 57 mg, Fiber: 2.7 g

Tuna Noodle Casserole

Preparation time: 10 minutes/**Cooking Time:** 45 minutes/**Total time:** 55 minutes

Servings: 6/**Difficulty Level:** Medium

Ingredients:

- 1 tablespoon olive oil
- 2 tablespoons flour
- 2 cups skim milk
- 1/4 cup low-fat cheddar cheese, shredded
- 3 cups cooked egg noodles
- 10-ounce package frozen peas, thawed
- 7 ounces' water-packed tuna
- 4 ounces' mushrooms, sliced
- 1/4 cup chopped green bell pepper
- l/s teaspoon black pepper
- 1/2 cup breadcrumbs

Instructions

Preheat oven to 375°F (190°C, or gas mark 5). Heat oil in a large skillet over low heat; add flour, stirring until smooth. Cook 1 minute, stirring constantly. Gradually add milk; cook over medium heat, constantly stirring, until mixture is thickened and bubbly. Stir in cheese; cook over low heat, constantly stirring, until cheese melts. Remove from heat. Combine cheese sauce, noodles, and the next 5 ingredients (black pepper). Spoon mixture into a 2-quart (1.9-L) casserole dish coated with nonstick vegetable oil spray. Sprinkle evenly with breadcrumbs. Bake for 35 minutes, or until the casserole is bubbly and the top is browned.

Nutritional Information: Calories: 277 kcal, protein: 19 g, carbohydrates: 40 g, Fat: 4 g, Cholesterol: 13 mg, Fiber: 7 g

Grill Mates Salmon with Eggplant and Zucchini

Preparation time: 10 minutes/**Cooking Time:** 30 minutes/**Total time:** 40 minutes

Servings: 1/**Difficulty Level:** Medium

Ingredients:

- 1 medium Zucchini; sliced
- 7 oz. Raw Salmon Filets
- 1 tsp of Pepper Seasoning
- 2 slices of Eggplant
- 1 can of Cooking spray
- 1/2 tsp of Black Pepper

Instructions

Preheat your outdoor grill to high. Coat the tin foil with the cooking spray. Sprinkle 1 tsp of pepper seasonings on the fillet. Place the salmon on a piece of tin foil large enough to cover around the fillet, skin side down. Join the longer sides of the foil together up and around the fish. To form a seal and prevent the fold from falling apart, fold the foil sides together.

Arrange the eggplant and zucchini slices in the grill basket. Sprinkle a pinch of black pepper (optional).

Close the grill cover after placing the salmon and grill basket with veggies on the grill. After 15 minutes, check the salmon for doneness; it will be done light pink. After 15 minutes, flip the veggies in the grill basket. Cook for another 10 minutes or until the veggies and fish are done.

Nutritional Information: Calories: 350 kcal, protein: 34.8 g, carbohydrates: 21.2 g, Fat: 17.3 g, Cholesterol: 66.3 mg, Fiber: 7 g

Baked Tilapia in Garlic and Olive Oil

Preparation time: 10 minutes plus marination time/**Cooking Time:** 30 minutes

Total time: 1 h/**Servings:** 4/**Difficulty Level:** Medium

Ingredients

- 4 cloves of crushed garlic
- 4 fillets of tilapia (4 ounces)
- 3 tablespoons of olive oil
- ¼ teaspoon of cayenne pepper
- 1 chopped onion,

Instructions

Place the fish fillets on a non-reactive shallow dish after rubbing them with crushed garlic. Drizzle the olive oil over the fish until evenly covered using a spoon. On top of the fish, place the onion. Let the fish marinate in the marinade overnight by covering it and refrigerating it.

Preheat an oven to 350°F (180°C) (175 degrees C). Transfer the fish and garlic, olive oil, and onion to a 9x13 inch baking dish. Season the fish with white pepper or cayenne pepper. Wrap the fish, onion, garlic, oil, and pepper in aluminum foil if you're grilling it and bake for 30 minutes.

Nutritional Information: Calories: 217 kcal, protein: 23.5 g, carbohydrates: 3.6 g, Fat: 11.7 g, Cholesterol: 41.5 mg, Fiber: 5 g

Greek Fish Stew

Preparation time: 5 minutes /**Cooking Time:** 25 minutes/**Total time:** 30 minutes

Servings: 4/**Difficulty Level:** Medium

Ingredients

- 4 ounces' orzo, or other small pasta
- 1/2 cup onion, chopped
- 1/2 teaspoon minced garlic
- 1 teaspoon fennel seed
- 2 cups canned no-salt-added tomatoes
- 2 cups low sodium chicken broth
- 1 tablespoon dried parsley
- 1/2 teaspoon black pepper
- 1/4 teaspoon turmeric
- 1 2 ounces' cod fillets, cut in 1 -inch (2.5-cm) cubes

Instructions

Cook pasta according to package directions. Drain and set aside. In a wide nonstick saucepan coated with a nonstick vegetable oil spray. Cook garlic, onions, and fennel seed until onion is tender. Add broth, tomatoes, parsley, pepper, and turmeric. Reduce heat and simmer for 10 minutes. Add fish and simmer for 5 minutes, or until fish is cooked through. Divide pasta among four bowls. Ladle soup over pasta.

Nutritional Information: Calories: 226 kcal, protein: 23 g, carbohydrates: 30 g, Fat: 2 g, Cholesterol: 37 mg, Fiber: 3 g

Sesame Fish

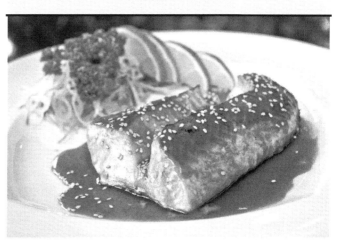

Preparation time: 40 minutes /**Cooking Time:** 20 minutes/**Total time:** 60 minutes

Servings: 4/**Difficulty Level:** Medium

Ingredients

- 1-pound halibut fillets
- 1/2 cup Reduced-Sodium Teriyaki Sauce
- 2 tablespoons sesame seeds
- 1 tablespoon flour
- 1/2 teaspoon white pepper

Instructions

Fill a shallow baking dish halfway with fillets. Pour teriyaki sauce on top of the fish. Refrigerate for 30 minutes or overnight if covered. Preheat the oven to 450 degrees Fahrenheit (230 degrees Celsius, or gas mark 8). Combine sesame seeds, flour, and pepper in a mixing bowl. Each fillet should be dipped in the flour mixture. Spray a nonstick baking pan using nonstick vegetable oil spray and arrange the fillets in a single layer on the pan. Using a nonstick vegetable oil spray, lightly coat the tops of each fillet and bake for 15 minutes, or till golden brown and the fish flakes readily when pierced with a fork.

Nutritional Information: Calories: 163 kcal, protein: 26 g, carbohydrates: 7 g, Fat: 3 g, Cholesterol: 36 mg, Fiber: 0 g

Orange Maple Glazed Salmon

Preparation time: 15 minutes /**Cooking Time:** 15 minutes/**Total time:** 30 minutes

Servings: 4/**Difficulty Level:** Medium

Ingredients

- 4 (4- to 6-ounce, 113 to 170 g) salmon fillets, pin bones removed
- ¼ cup pure maple syrup
- juice of 2 oranges
- zest of 1 orange
- 2 tbsps. low-sodium soy sauce
- 1 tsp. garlic powder

Instructions

Preheat the oven to 400°F(205°C). Add the maple syrup, orange juice and zest, soy sauce, and garlic powder into a small, shallow dish, whisk them together well. Flesh-side down to put the salmon pieces into the dish. Allow it to marinate for 10 minutes. Then skin-side up to transfer the salmon to a rimmed baking sheet, bake until the flesh is opaque, about 15 minutes.

Nutritional Information: Calories: 297 kcal, protein: 34 g, carbohydrates: 18 g, Fat: 11 g, Cholesterol: 3 mg, Fiber: less than 1 g

Haddock Tacos with Cabbage

Preparation time: 10 minutes /**Cooking Time:** 5 minutes/**Total time:** 20 minutes

Servings: 4/**Difficulty Level:** Medium

Ingredients

- 8 ounces (227 g) skinless haddock fillets, cut into 1-inch chunks

- 2 cups angel hair cabbage
- 2 tbsps. fresh lime juice
- 3 tsps. extra-virgin olive oil
- 2 (6-inch) whole-wheat tortillas, warmed
- 1 tsp. of ground cumin
- ⅛ tsp. salt
- ½ tsp. of chili powder
- ½ avocado, chopped
- ⅛ tsp. black pepper; freshly ground
- Fresh cilantro

Instructions

Mix the chili powder, cumin, salt, and pepper in a small bowl. Add the haddock and toss to coat. Mix the cabbage, lime juice, avocado, and 1 tsp in a small bowl. Olive oil. Heat the remaining olive oil in a medium skillet over medium to high heat. Add the haddock and cook for 4 to 5 minutes, turning until the fish is opaque and flakes easily with a fork. Portion the fish between the warmed tortillas and top with the cabbage avocado mixture. Serve topped with fresh cilantro.

Nutritional Information: Calories: 368 kcal, protein: 32 g, carbohydrates: 22 g, Fat: 16 g, Cholesterol: 84 mg, Fiber: 7 g

Pecan-Crusted Catfish

Preparation time: 5 minutes /**Cooking Time:** 12 minutes/**Total time:** 20 minutes

Servings: 4/**Difficulty Level:** Easy

Ingredients

- 6 tablespoons Dijon mustard
- 1/4 cup skim milk
- 1 cup pecans, ground
-
- 1-pound catfish fillets

Instructions

Preheat oven to 450°F (230°C, or gas mark 8). Coat a baking sheet with nonstick vegetable oil spray. Mix mustard and milk in a shallow dish. Spread pecans in another dish. Dip fillets in mustard mixture, then roll in pecans to coat. Place on prepared pan. Bake 10 to 12 minutes, or until fish flakes easily.

Nutritional Information: Calories: 364 kcal, protein: 22 g, carbohydrates: 6 g, Fat: 29 g,

Cholesterol: 54 mg, Fiber: 3 g

Brown Rice Tuna Bake

Preparation time: 10 minutes /**Cooking Time:** 60 minutes/**Total time:** 1 hour 10 minutes/**Servings:** 6/**Difficulty Level:** Easy

Ingredients

- 1 1/4 cups uncooked brown rice
- 3 cups water
- 1 cup chopped celery
- 1/2 cup onion, finely diced
- 1/2 cup plain fat-free yogurt
- 1 cup skim milk
- 1/4 teaspoon red pepper flakes
- 1/2 teaspoon dried tarragon
- 14 ounces' water-packed canned tuna, drained
- 2 cups frozen peas, thawed
- 3/4 cup low-fat cheddar cheese, shredded

Instructions

Preheat oven to 350°F (180°C, or gas mark 4). Combine rice and water in a large saucepan. Bring to a boil. Reduce heat, cover, and cook for 35 minutes. Remove from heat. Add celery, onion, yogurt, and milk. Add red pepper flakes and tarragon; mix well. Flake the tuna with a fork, add it, and thaw peas to the rice mixture; mix well. Pour into 2-quart (1.9-L) casserole dish. Bake for 30 minutes. Top with shredded cheese.

Nutritional Information: Calories: 321 kcal, protein: 29 g, carbohydrates: 42 g, Fat: 3 g, Cholesterol: 25 mg, Fiber: 4 g

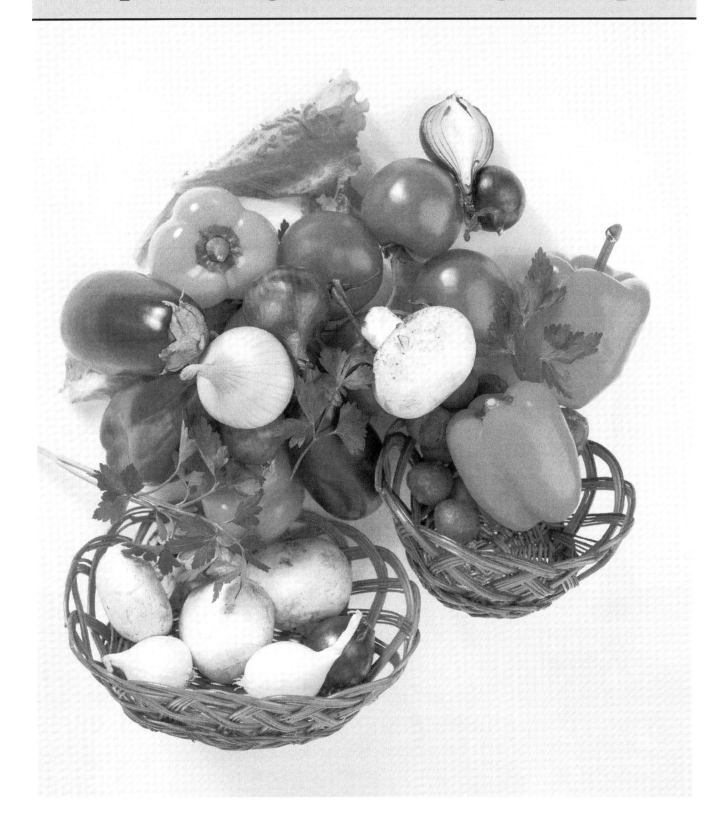

Roasted Root Veggies and Spiced Lentils

Preparation time: 5 minutes/**Cooking Time:** 45 minutes/**Total time:** 50 minutes

Servings: 4/**Difficulty Level:** Easy

Ingredients:

Lentils

- ½ cup of French green lentils or black beluga lentils
- 1 ½ cups of water
- ½ teaspoon of ground coriander
- 1 teaspoon of garlic powder
- ¼ teaspoon of ground allspice
- ½ teaspoon of ground cumin
- ¼ teaspoon of kosher salt
- 1 teaspoon of olive oil; extra-virgin
- 2 tablespoons of lemon juice

Vegetables

- 1 1/2 cups of roasted root vegetables
- 1 smashed clove of garlic,
- 2 cups of chopped beet greens or kale
- ⅛ teaspoon of ground pepper
- 1 teaspoon of ground coriander
- 1 tablespoon of olive oil; extra-virgin
- dash of kosher salt
- For garnish; fresh parsley
- 2 tablespoons of plain low-fat yogurt or tahini

Instructions

To make lentils: In a medium saucepan, mix the lentils, water, garlic powder, cumin, 1/4 teaspoon of salt, allspice, 1/2 teaspoon of coriander, and sumac (if using). Boil it. Reduce heat to keep the simmer, cover, and cook for 25 to 30 minutes. Uncover and continue to cook for another 5 minutes, or until the liquid has somewhat reduced. Drain. Add one teaspoon of oil and lemon juice.

Meanwhile, prepare the veggies: Heat the oil over medium heat in a large skillet. Add garlic and cook for 1 to 2 minutes, or until garlic is aromatic. Add roasted vegetables and cook, often turning, until vegetables are cooked through, for 2 to 4 minutes. Add and cook kale for 2 to 3 minutes, or until kale is barely wilted. Add the pepper, coriander, and salt and mix well. Serve the veggies over the lentils with a dollop of tahini on top (or yogurt). If desired, garnish with parsley.

Nutritional Information: Calories: 453 kcal, protein: 18.1 g, carbohydrates: 49.7 g, Fat: 22.4 g, Cholesterol: 8.3 mg, Fiber: 5 g

Tomato and Basil Quiche

Preparation time: 10 minutes/**Cooking Time:** 40 minutes/**Total time:** 50 minutes

Servings: 4/**Difficulty Level:** Easy

Ingredients:

- 2 cups of tomatoes, sliced
- 1 tablespoon of olive oil
- 2 tablespoons of flour
- 1 cup onion, sliced
- 2 teaspoons of dried basil
- 1/2 cup skim milk
- 3/4 cup egg substitute
- 1/2 teaspoon black pepper
- 1 cup Swiss cheese, shredded

Instructions

Preheat the oven to 400 degrees Fahrenheit (200 degrees Celsius, or gas mark 6). In a large skillet, heat the olive oil over medium heat. Remove onion from skillet when it has softened. Cook for 1 minute on each side after sprinkling tomato slices with flour and basil. Whisk together the egg substitute and milk in a small bowl. Season with salt and pepper. Half of the cheese should be spread in the bottom of a pie pan that has been coated with nonstick vegetable oil. Onions should be layered on top of the cheese, and tomatoes should be on top of that. Over the vegetables, pour the egg mixture. The remaining cheese should be sprinkled on top. 10 minutes in the oven Bake for 15 to 20 minutes, or until the filling is puffy and golden brown, at 350°F (180°C, or gas mark 4). Warm the dish before serving.

Nutritional Information: Calories: 188 kcal, protein: 18 g, carbohydrates: 14 g, Fat: 7 g, Cholesterol:13 mg, Fiber: 2 g

Vegetarian Bolognese

Preparation time: 10 minutes/**Cooking Time:** 4 hours 20 minutes/**Total time:** 4 hours 30 minutes/**Servings:** 8/**Difficulty Level:** Medium

Ingredients:

- ½ cup of dry white wine
- 1 (28 ounces) can have diced San Marzano tomatoes,
- ½ cup of vegetable broth; low-sodium or water
- ½ cup of chopped celery
- 1 cup of chopped onion
- 3 tablespoons of olive oil; extra-virgin
- ½ cup of chopped carrot
- 1 teaspoon of Italian seasoning
- 2 tablespoons of minced garlic
- ¼ teaspoon of ground pepper
- ½ teaspoon of salt
- ¼ cup of heavy cream
- ¼ cup of chopped fresh basil.
- 2 (15 ounces) cans of cannellini beans; no-salt-added or rinsed small white beans,
- ½ cup of grated Parmesan cheese
- 1 pound of whole-wheat spaghetti

Instructions

In a 5- to the 6-quart slow cooker, add wine, tomatoes, onion, celery, carrot, oil, garlic, broth (or water), salt, Italian seasoning, and pepper. Cook for 4 hours on high or 8 hours on low. At the end of the cooking time, add the cream and beans. Keep it warm. Bring a big saucepan of water to a boil in the meanwhile. Drain pasta after cooking according to package instructions. Using 8 bowls, divide the spaghetti. Add the Parmesan, sauce, and basil to the top.

Nutritional Information: Calories: 434 kcal, protein: 15.9 g, carbohydrates: 64.3 g, Fat: 12.6 g, Cholesterol:12.1 mg, Fiber: 4 g

Broccoli Wild Rice Casserole

Preparation time: 10 minutes/**Cooking Time:** 60 minutes/**Total time:** 1 hour 10 minutes/**Servings:** 6/**Difficulty Level:** Easy

Ingredients:

- 1 1/2 cups wild rice
- 6 cups broccoli
- 2 cups reduced-sodium cream of mushroom soup
- 2 cups low fat cheddar cheese, shredded

Instructions

Preheat the oven to 325°F (170°C, or gas mark 3) before starting. Prepare wild rice as directed on the package. In the bottom of a 9 × 9-inch (23 x 23-cm) casserole pan, layer rice. Broccoli should be steamed for 5 minutes before being layered on top of rice. Toss the soup with the cheese and distribute it on top of the broccoli. Bake for 45 minutes, uncovered.

Nutritional Information: Calories: 293 kcal, protein: 20 g, carbohydrates: 44 g, Fat: 5 g, Cholesterol:12 mg, Fiber: 5 g

Grilled Eggplant and Tomato Pasta

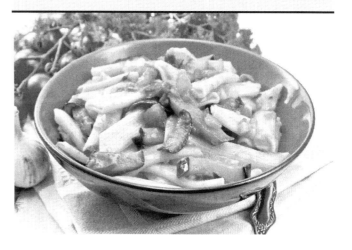

Preparation time: 5 minutes/**Cooking Time:** 25 minutes/**Total time:** 30 minutes

Servings: 4/**Difficulty Level:** Medium

Ingredients:

- 2 teaspoons of chopped fresh oregano.

- 4 tablespoons of olive oil; extra-virgin, divided.
- 1 pound of chopped plum tomatoes,
- ½ teaspoon of ground pepper
- 1 grated clove of garlic,
- ½ teaspoon of salt
- ¼ teaspoon of crushed red pepper
- ½ cup of chopped fresh basil.
- 1 ½ pound of eggplant, 1/2-inch-thick slices
- ¼ cup of crumbled feta cheese or shaved Ricotta Salata
- 8 ounces of whole-wheat penne

Instructions

Bring a big saucepan of water to a boil. Preheat the grill to medium-high heat. In a large mixing bowl, combine 3 tablespoons of oil, crushed red pepper, tomatoes, garlic, pepper, oregano, and salt. Brush the remaining one tablespoon of oil over the eggplant. Grill for 4 minutes on each side, flipping once until cooked and browned in places. Allow 10 minutes for cooling. Chop them into bite-size pieces and add to the tomatoes with basils. In the meanwhile, prepare the pasta according to the package instructions. Drain. Toss the tomato mixture with the spaghetti and serve. Cheese should be sprinkled on top.

Nutritional Information: Calories: 449 kcal, protein: 13.5 g, carbohydrates: 62.1 g, Fat: 19.2 g, Cholesterol: 8.3 mg, Fiber: 3 g

Potato and Winter Vegetable Casserole

Preparation time: 10 minutes/**Cooking Time:** 30 minutes/**Total time:** 40 minutes

Servings: 6/**Difficulty Level:** Medium

Ingredients:

- 6 potatoes
- 2 tablespoons olive oil
- 1 cup onion, sliced
- 2 cups cabbage, chopped
- 2 cups cauliflower, chopped
- 1 teaspoon garlic, crushed
- 1 cup plain fat-free yogurt
- 2 cups canned white kidney beans
- 1/4 cup fresh dill, chopped
- 1/2 teaspoon paprika

Instructions

Preheat oven to 325°F (170°C, or gas mark 3). Boil or microwave the potatoes until nearly done. When cool enough, peel if desired. Heat the olive oil in a large skillet over medium-high heat. Sauté the onions until soft. Add the cabbage, cauliflower, garlic, and fry until the cabbage and cauliflower are tender. Add the yogurt to the vegetable mixture. Drain and rinse the white beans and add to the vegetable mixture. Mix thoroughly and set aside. Slice the potatoes into rounds and put half the slices on the bottom of a 9 x 13-inch (23 x 33-cm) baking dish sprayed with nonstick vegetable oil. Spread the vegetable mixture over the potatoes. Cover with the remaining potatoes. Sprinkle with dill and paprika. Bake for 20 minutes.

Nutritional Information: Calories: 462 kcal, protein: 17 g, carbohydrates: 88 g, Fat: 6 g, Cholesterol: 1 mg, Fiber: 12 g

Rainbow Grain Bowl and Cashew Tahini Sauce

Preparation time: 20 minutes/**Cooking Time:** 0 minutes/**Total time:** 20 minutes

Servings: 1/**Difficulty Level:** Medium

Ingredients:

- ¼ cup of packed parsley leaves
- ½ cup of water
- ¼ teaspoon of salt
- 1 tablespoon of cider vinegar or lemon juice
- ½ teaspoon of tamari or soy sauce; extra-virgin
- ¾ cup of unsalted cashews
- ½ cup of cooked lentils
- 1 tablespoon of olive oil; extra-virgin
- ¼ cup of grated raw beet
- ½ cup of cooked quinoa
- ¼ cup of chopped bell pepper
- ½ cup of shredded red cabbage
- ¼ cup of grated carrot
- For garnish,1 tablespoon of chopped Toasted cashews.
- ¼ cup of sliced cucumber

Instructions

Mix water, tamari (or soy sauce), cashews, lemon juice (or vinegar), oil, parsley, and salt in a blender. In the middle of a shallow serving dish, combine lentils and quinoa. Cabbage, carrot, beet, pepper, and cucumber go on top. Two tablespoons of cashew sauce are spooned over the top (save the extra sauce for another use). If desired, garnish with cashews.

Nutritional Information: Calories: 361 kcal, protein: 16.6 g, carbohydrates: 53.9 g, Fat: 10.1 g, Cholesterol: 1 mg, Fiber: 6 g

Mexican Bean Bake

Preparation time: 5 minutes/**Cooking Time:** 20 minutes/**Total time:** 25 minutes

Servings: 6/**Difficulty Level:** Medium

Ingredients:

- 2 cups refried beans
- 4 cups cooked rice
- 2 cups canned black beans, drained
- 1 cup salsa
- 1 cup low-fat cheddar cheese, shredded

Instructions

Preheat oven to 375°F (190°C, or gas mark 5). In a 9 x 9-inch (23 x 23-cm) baking dish, spread out the refried beans. Layer cooked rice on top. Layer black beans on top of rice. Spread with salsa. Sprinkle with cheese. Bake for 15 to 20 minutes, or until heated through and cheese is melted.

Nutritional Information: Calories: 334 kcal, protein: 19 g, carbohydrates: 57 g, Fat: 3 g, Cholesterol: 11 mg, Fiber: 11 g

Chickpea and Potato Curry

Preparation time: 5 minutes/**Cooking Time:** 30 minutes/**Total time:** 35 minutes

Servings: 15/**Difficulty Level:** Medium

Ingredients:

- 3 tablespoons of canola oil or grapeseed oil
- 1 pound of peeled Yukon Gold potatoes, 1-inch pieces
- 3 minced cloves of garlic,
- 1 large, diced onion,

- ¾ teaspoon of salt
- 2 teaspoons of curry powder
- 1 (14 ounces) can have diced tomatoes; no-salt-added
- ¼ teaspoon of cayenne pepper
- 1 (15 ounces) can of chickpeas, low-sodium, rinsed
- ¾ cup of water, divided.
- ½ teaspoon of garam masala
- 1 cup of frozen peas

Instructions

In a large saucepan with a steamer basket, boil 1 inch of water. Add the potatoes, cover, and steam for 6 to 8 minutes, or until tender. Remove the potatoes and set them aside. Dry the pan.

In a medium-high-heat saucepan, heat the oil. Add onion and cook, often turning, until the onion is tender and transparent, for 3 to 5 minutes. Add and cook salt, curry powder, garlic, and cayenne, stirring continuously, for 1 minute, until fragrant. Cook for 2 minutes after adding the tomatoes and their juice. Fill a blender or food processor halfway with the mixture. Puree with 1/2 cup water until smooth.

Put the purée back in the saucepan. To rinse the sauce residue, pulse with the remaining 1/4 cup of water in the blender or food processor. Add the peas, chickpeas, saved potatoes, and gram masala to the pot. Cook for 5 minutes, often stirring, until heated.

Gram masala, a spice blend of coriander, cumin, black pepper, cinnamon, cardamom, and other spices, gives this Indian stew a warming, rich layer of flavor.

Nutritional Information: Calories: 321 kcal, protein: 8.9 g, carbohydrates: 46.5 g, Fat: 11.5 g, Cholesterol: 3.8 mg, Fiber: 6 g

Squash and Rice Bake

Preparation time: 5 minutes/**Cooking Time:** 40 minutes/**Total time:** 45 minutes

Servings: 4/**Difficulty Level:** Medium

Ingredients:

- 1/2 cup rice
- 2 tablespoons olive oil

- 1/4 teaspoon minced garlic
- 1/2 teaspoon dried thyme
- 4 cups yellow squash, sliced
- 2 ounces' low-fat Swiss cheese, shredded

Instructions

Preheat oven to 350°F (180°C, or gas mark 4). Cook rice according to package directions. Heat oil in a large skillet. Sauté garlic for a few minutes. Add thyme and squash. Sauté for a few minutes more. Stir the rice and cheese into the mixture. Turn into a 2-quart (1.9-L) baking dish that has been coated with nonstick vegetable oil spray. Bake for 25 minutes or until heated through.

Nutritional Information: Calories: 128 kcal, protein: 6 g, carbohydrates: 10 g, Fat: 8 g, Cholesterol: 5 mg, Fiber: 1 g

Zucchini Frittata

Preparation time: 10 minutes/**Cooking Time:** 20 minutes7**Total time:** 30 minutes

Servings: 4/**Difficulty Level:** Medium

Ingredients:

- 2 cups shredded zucchini
- 2 tablespoons olive oil
- 1/2 cup mushrooms, sliced
- 1 cup egg substitute
- 1/3 cup Swiss cheese, shredded

Instructions

Place the zucchini in a paper towel and squeeze out any excess moisture. Heat oil in a 10-inch (25-cm) skillet. Sauté the mushrooms briefly, then add the zucchini. Cook for 4 minutes, or until the squash is barely tender. Pour egg substitute over vegetables. Stir once quickly to coat vegetables. Cook over low heat until eggs begin to set. Sprinkle with the cheese. Place under the broiler until cheese browns. Let set for 2 to 3 minutes. Cut into wedges and serve.

Nutritional Information: Calories: 144 kcal, protein: 12 g, carbohydrates: 3 g, Fat: 10 g, Cholesterol: 4 mg, Fiber: 1 g

Carrot Rice

Preparation time: 10 minutes/**Cooking Time:** 40 minutes/**Total time:** 50 minutes

Servings: 6/**Difficulty Level:** Easy

Ingredients:

- 2 cups of water
- 1 cup of basmati rice
- 1 tablespoon of margarine
- ¼ cup of roasted peanuts
- 1 sliced onion,
- ¾ cup of grated carrots
- 1 teaspoon of fresh minced ginger root
- salt to taste
- fresh chopped cilantro
- cayenne pepper; to taste.

Instructions

In a medium saucepan, combine rice and water. Over high heat, bring to a boil. Reduce the heat to low, cover with a lid, and steam for 20 minutes, or until soft.

Grind the peanuts in a blender and put them aside. In a skillet, melt the margarine over medium heat. Add onion and cook, constantly stirring, for approximately 10 minutes, or until the onion is cooked and become golden brown. Add the ginger, carrots, and salt to taste. Reduce heat to low and cover for 5 minutes to steam. Add the peanuts and cayenne pepper and mix well. When the rice is done, pour it into the pan and gently mix it with the other ingredients. Serve with chopped cilantro as a garnish.

Nutritional Information: Calories: 179 kcal, protein: 4 g, carbohydrates: 30.1 g, Fat: 4.8 g, Cholesterol: 3 mg, Fiber: 2 g

Lentils and Pasta

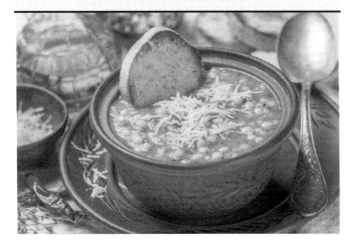

Preparation time: 10 minutes/**Cooking Time:** 60 minutes/**Total time:** 1 hour 10 minutes/**Servings:** 6/**Difficulty Level:** Easy

Ingredients:

- 1 cup lentils
- 1/2 cup celery, sliced
- 1 1/2 cups onion, coarsely chopped, divided
- 2 tablespoons olive oil
- 1/2 teaspoon cumin
- 1 tablespoon cilantro
- 6 ounces' fresh spinach
- 8 ounces' pasta (small shapes like orzo are best)

Instructions

Cook lentils in 6 cups (1.4 L) water with celery and 1 1/2 cups (80 g) of the onion until soft, about 40 minutes. Heat the olive oil and sauté the remaining onions, cumin, and cilantro until the onions are soft in a large skillet. Add spinach and sauté until wilted, another 4 to 5 minutes. Drain lentils and stir into the onion-spinach mixture. Cook pasta according to package directions. Stir into mixture.

Nutritional Information: Calories: 245 kcal, protein: 10 g, carbohydrates: 40 g, Fat: 5 g, Cholesterol: 0 mg, Fiber: 6 g

Cheese Pie

Preparation time: 10 minutes/**Cooking Time:** 40 minutes/**Total time:** 50 minutes

Servings: 4/**Difficulty Level:** Easy

Ingredients:

- 4 ounces feta cheese
- 16 ounces' low fat ricotta cheese
- 1 cup egg substitute
- 1/4 cup flour
- 3/4 cup skim milk
- 1/4 teaspoon black pepper

Instructions

Preheat oven to 375°F (190°C, or gas mark 5). Spray an ovenproof skillet or glass baking dish with nonstick vegetable oil spray. Mix the cheeses, then stir in the egg substitute, flour, milk, and pepper. Pour the batter into the prepared pan. Bake for 40 minutes, or until golden and set. Cut into wedges.

Nutritional Information: Calories: 332 kcal, protein: 27 g, carbohydrates: 16 g, Fat: 17 g, Cholesterol: 62 mg, Fiber: 0 g

Veggie and Hummus Sandwich

Preparation time: 10 minutes/**Cooking Time:** 0 minutes/**Total time:** 10 minutes

Servings: 1/**Difficulty Level:** Easy

Ingredients:

- ¼ medium sliced red bell pepper,
- 2 slices of whole-grain bread
- ¼ cup of sliced cucumber
- ½ cup of mixed salad greens
- ¼ cup of shredded carrot
- 3 tablespoons of hummus
- ¼ mashed avocado,

Instructions

Spread hummus on one piece of bread and avocado on the other. Greens, cucumber, bell pepper, and carrot are placed in the sandwich. Serve by slicing in half.

Nutritional Information: Calories: 325 kcal, protein: 12.8 g, carbohydrates: 39.7 g, Fat: 14.3 g, Cholesterol: 0 mg, Fiber: 1 g

Pasta primavera

Preparation time: 10 minutes/**Cooking Time:** 30 minutes/**Total time:** 40 minutes

Servings: 6/**Difficulty Level:** Easy

Ingredients:

- 1 cup of sliced yellow squash or zucchini
- 1 cup of sliced mushrooms
- 2 cups of broccoli florets
- 1 tablespoon of olive oil; extra-virgin
- 2 cups of sliced green or red peppers
- 2 minced garlic cloves,
- 1/2 cup of chopped onion
- 1 cup of evaporated fat-free milk
- 1 teaspoon of butter
- 3/4 cup of Parmesan cheese; freshly grated.
- 1/3 cup of fresh finely chopped parsley.
- 12 ounces of whole-wheat pasta

Instructions

Bring 1 inch of water to a boil in a big saucepan with a steamer basket. Add mushrooms, zucchini, broccoli, and peppers. Cover and steam for 10 minutes, or until tender-crisp. Remove the saucepan from the heat.

Heat the olive oil in a wide saucepan and sauté the garlic and onion over medium heat. Stir or shake the steamed veggies to evenly cover them in the garlic and onion mixture. Remove the pan from the heat but keep it warm.

Heat the milk, butter, and Parmesan cheese in a separate wide pot. Stir constantly over low heat until the sauce has thickened and cooked thoroughly. Stir constantly to avoid scalding. Remove the pan from the heat but keep it warm.

Fill a big saucepan 3/4 full of water and bring to a boil in the meanwhile. Cook pasta for 10 to 12 minutes, or according to package instructions, until the pasta is al dente (tender). Drain all of the water from the pasta.

Distribute the spaghetti equally among the plates. Pour the sauce over the after topping with vegetables. Serve immediately with fresh parsley as a garnish.

Nutritional Information: Calories: 347 kcal, protein: 17 g, carbohydrates: 54 g, Fat: 7 g, Cholesterol: 12 mg, Fiber: 4 g

Pizza Omelet

Preparation time: 10 minutes/**Cooking Time:** 10 minutes/**Total time:** 20 minutes

Servings: 2/**Difficulty Level:** Easy

Ingredients:

- 1 cup egg substitute
- 2 tablespoons fat-free sour cream
- 2 tablespoons water
- 1/2 teaspoon Italian seasoning
- 1/2 cup mushrooms, sliced
- 1/4 cup onion, sliced
- 1/4 cup green bell pepper, coarsely chopped
- 1/4 cup spaghetti sauce, heated
- 2 ounces part-skim mozzarella, shredded

Instructions

Whisk together egg substitute, sour cream, water, and Italian seasoning until fluffy. Sauté mushrooms, onion, and green bell pepper until onion becomes soft. Pour egg mixture into a heated nonstick skillet or omelet pan sprayed with nonstick vegetable oil spray. Lift the edges as it cooks to allow uncooked egg to run underneath. Cover half the omelet with the vegetables and fold the other half over the top when it is nearly set. Remove to plate. Top with heated sauce and cheese.

Nutritional Information: Calories: 232 kcal, protein: 24 g, carbohydrates: 9 g, Fat: 9 g, Cholesterol: 25 mg, Fiber: 2 g

Vegetarian chili and tofu

Preparation time: 5 minutes/**Cooking Time:** 35 minutes/**Total time:** 40 minutes

Servings: 4/**Difficulty Level:** Easy

Ingredients:

- 12 ounces of extra-firm tofu; small pieces
- 1 small chopped yellow onion (1/2 cup)
- 1 no salt added, can of kidney beans; rinsed and drained (14 ounces)
- 2 no added salt cans of diced tomatoes (14 ounces each)
- 1 tablespoon of olive oil

- 3 tablespoons of chili powder
- 1 no salt added can of black beans; rinsed and drained (14 ounces)
- 1 tablespoon of chopped fresh cilantro.
- 1 tablespoon of oregano

Instructions

Heat olive oil in a soup pot over medium heat. Add onions and cook for approximately 6 minutes, or until tender and transparent. Add tomatoes, tofu, chili powder, beans, and oregano. Cook it. Reduce the heat to low and cook for at least 30 minutes. Take the pan off the heat and toss in the cilantro. Immediately ladle into separate bowls and serve.

Nutritional Information: Calories: 314 kcal, protein: 19 g, carbohydrates: 46 g, Fat: 6 g, Cholesterol: 0 mg, Fiber: 4 g

Spinach-Stuffed Tomatoes

Preparation time: 10 minutes/**Cooking Time:** 20 minutes/**Total time:** 30 minutes

Servings: 4/**Difficulty Level:** Medium

Ingredients:

- 10 ounces fresh spinach
- 4 tomatoes
- 1 cup part-skim mozzarella, divided
- 1/4 cup onion, finely chopped
- 1/4 cup Parmesan, grated
- l/s teaspoon pepper
- 2 tablespoons fresh parsley, minced

Instructions

Preheat oven to 350°F (180°C, or gas mark 4). Steam spinach or microwave in a covered bowl until softened but still slightly crispy. Drain well and squeeze dry. Put in a large bowl. Remove the pulp from the tomatoes after slicing and hollowing them out. Seeds should be discarded. Finely chop the pulp and toss it in with the spinach. Blend spinach with 11/2 cup of mozzarella cheese, Parmesan, onion, and pepper. Fill tomato shells with the mixture. The remaining mozzarella & parsley should be sprinkled over the top. Bake for 6 minutes, or till heated through, in an 8-inch (20-cm) round glass or ceramic baking dish.

Nutritional Information: Calories: 158 kcal, protein: 14 g, carbohydrates: 13 g, Fat: 7 g, Cholesterol: 24 mg, Fiber: 4 g

Bean and Tomato Curry

Preparation time: 10 minutes/**Cooking Time:** 20 minutes/**Total time:** 30 minutes

Servings: 6/**Difficulty Level:** Medium

Ingredients:

- 1 tablespoon canola oil
- 1 teaspoon mustard seed
- 1 teaspoon cumin seeds
- 1 cup onion, chopped
- 1 tablespoon fresh ginger, peeled and chopped
- 1/2 teaspoon chopped garlic
- 4 cups canned no-salt-added tomatoes
- 2 cups kidney beans, drained and rinsed
- 1 teaspoon curry powder

Instructions

Heat oil in a large pot over medium heat and stir-fry the mustard and cumin seeds until they pop. Add onion, ginger, and garlic, and stir-fry until lightly colored. Add tomatoes with juice, beans, and curry powder. Simmer for about 20 minutes or until thick and saucy.

Nutritional Information: Calories: 140 kcal, protein: 7 g, carbohydrates: 23 g, Fat: 3 g, Cholesterol: 0 mg, Fiber: 6 g

Garbanzo Curry

Preparation time: 10 minutes/**Cooking Time:** 4-5 hours/**Total time:** 5 hours 10 minutes/**Servings:** 4/**Difficulty Level:** Easy

Ingredients:

- 2 tablespoons canola oil
- 1 cup onion, diced
- 1/2 teaspoon minced garlic
- 1 teaspoon fresh ginger, peeled and grated
- 1 teaspoon cumin
- 1 teaspoon coriander
- 1 teaspoon turmeric

- 2 cups canned garbanzo beans, drained and rinsed
- 2 cups canned no-salt-added tomatoes
- 1/2 teaspoon garam masala

Instructions

Heat oil in a heavy skillet. Sauté onion, garlic, ginger, cumin, coriander, and turmeric until soft onion. Place onion mixture and remaining ingredients in a slow cooker and cook on low for 8 to 10 hours or on high for 4 to 5 hours.

Nutritional Information: Calories: 246 kcal, protein: 8 g, carbohydrates: 37 g, Fat: 9 g, Cholesterol: 0 mg, Fiber: 7 g

Tofu and Broccoli Stir-Fry

Preparation time: 10 minutes/**Cooking Time:** 20 minutes/**Total time:** 30 minutes

Servings: 4/**Difficulty Level:** Easy

Ingredients:

- 1 2 ounces firm tofu
- 6 tablespoons Reduced-Sodium Soy Sauce
- 2 tablespoons mirin wine
- 1 teaspoon sesame oil
- 1/4 teaspoon minced garlic
- 1/2 teaspoon ground ginger
- 1 tablespoon olive oil
- 6 cups broccoli florets
- 1/2 cup mushrooms, sliced

Instructions

Remove tofu from package and drain under a plate or other weight. Combine soy sauce, mirin, sesame oil, garlic, and ginger. Remove tofu from weight, cut into 3f4-inch (2-cm) cubes, and place in soy sauce mixture. Heat olive oil in a wok or large skillet. Stir-fry broccoli and mushrooms until broccoli is crisp-tender. Remove from wok. Add tofu and cook until it turns golden, then carefully cook the other sides. Return vegetables to wok. Add remaining marinade. Cook and stir carefully until heated through.

Nutritional Information: Calories: 155 kcal, protein: 9 g, carbohydrates: 156 g, Fat: 7 g,

Cholesterol: 0 mg, Fiber: 0 g

Corn Chowder

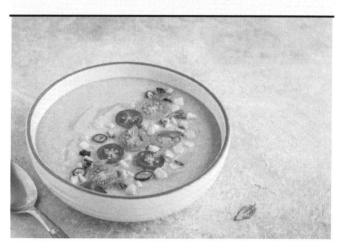

Preparation time: 5 minutes/**Cooking Time:** 30 minutes/**Total time:** 35 minutes

Servings: 6/**Difficulty Level:** Medium

Ingredients:

- 1 tablespoon olive oil
- 1 cup onion, chopped
- 1/2 cup celery, sliced
- 1/2 cup carrot, sliced
- 2 tablespoons flour
- 2 cups low sodium chicken broth
- 4 cups skim milk
- 2 potatoes, peeled and diced
- 3 cups frozen corn, thawed
- 1/2 teaspoon black pepper

Instructions

Heat the oil in a large Dutch oven. Add the onion, celery, and carrots and cook over medium heat until soft. Sprinkle on the flour and cook for 3 minutes, stirring frequently. Stir in the broth and milk. Add the potatoes and corn. Simmer for 25 minutes or until potatoes are tender. Sprinkle with pepper.

Nutritional Information: Calories: 278 kcal, protein: 13 g, carbohydrates: 52 g, Fat: 4 g, Cholesterol: 3 mg, Fiber: 5 g

Southwestern vegan bowl

Preparation time: 5 minutes/**Cooking Time:** 55 minutes/**Total time:** 60 minutes

Servings: 6/**Difficulty Level:** Medium

Ingredients:

- 1 cup of chopped red onion.
- 2 teaspoons of canola oil
- 2 cups of green bell pepper; chopped.
- 1 cup of diced sweet potato
- 1 minced chili pepper
- 2 minced cloves of garlic,
- 1 cup of chopped tomato
- 1/2 cup of green lentils
- 1 cup of brown rice
- 1 tablespoon of ground cumin
- 1/2 cup of red lentils
- 2 cups of vegetable stock; no-salt-added.
- 1 tablespoon of fresh ground pepper
- 4 cups of chopped kale
- 1 tablespoon of red wine vinegar
- 2 cups of water
- 1 cup of cooked black beans
- 4 lime wedges
- 2 tablespoons of minced fresh cilantro

Instructions

Heat canola oil in a large sauté pan over medium-high heat. Add garlic, onion, sweet potato, peppers, and tomato. Cook for 10-15 mins, or until the onions are transparent.

Add lentils, stock, rice, vinegar, spices, and water. Bring to a boil, then lower the heat. Cook for about 45 minutes with the lid on. Toss with black beans, kale, and cilantro before serving. Serve with lime wedges as a garnish.

Nutritional Information: Calories: 376 kcal, protein: 18 g, carbohydrates: 68 g, Fat: 4 g, Cholesterol: 0 mg, Fiber: 2 g

Polenta with vegetables

Preparation time: 5 minutes/**Cooking Time:** 55 minutes/**Total time:** 60 minutes

Servings: 4/**Difficulty Level:** Medium

Ingredients:

- 4 cups of water
- 1 cup of cornmeal (polenta); coarsely ground.
- 1 cup of fresh mushrooms; sliced.
- 1 teaspoon of chopped garlic,
- 1 cup of broccoli florets
- 1 cup of sliced onions
- 1 cup of sliced zucchini
- Chopped basil, fresh oregano, or rosemary to taste.
- 2 tablespoons of Parmesan cheese; grated.

Instructions

Preheat an oven to 350 degrees Fahrenheit. Spray a 3-quart ovenproof dish lightly with cooking spray. In the prepared dish, add water, polenta, and garlic. Bake it, uncovered, for approximately 40 minutes, or until the polenta peels away from the edges of the baking dish. The polenta must be moist. Spray a nonstick pan with the cooking spray while the polenta is cooking. Add onions and mushrooms. Cook, occasionally stirring, until the veggies are cooked, approximately 5 minutes.

Boil 1 inch of water in a saucepan with a steamer basket. Add zucchini and broccoli. Cover and steam for 2 to 3 minutes, or until tender-crisp. Top the polenta with the cooked veggies when it's done. Top with cheese and herbs. Serve right away.

Nutritional Information: Calories: 178 kcal, protein: 6 g, carbohydrates: 34 g, Fat: 1 g, Cholesterol: 2 mg, Fiber: 4 g

Fresh puttanesca & brown rice

Preparation time: 5 minutes/**Cooking Time:** 35 minutes/**Total time:** 40 minutes

Servings: 4/**Difficulty Level:** Medium

Ingredients:

- 1 tablespoon of minced garlic
- 4 cups of ripe chopped plum tomatoes
- 1 1/2 tablespoons of capers; rinsed and drained
- 1/4 cup of fresh chopped basil
- 4 pitted and sliced Kalamata olives,
- 1 tablespoon of olive oil
- 4 pitted and sliced green olives,

- 1 tablespoon of fresh minced parsley
- 3 cups of cooked brown rice
- 1/8 teaspoon of red pepper flakes

Instructions

Combine the olives, garlic, tomatoes, capers, and oil in a large mixing basin. Stir in the parsley, basil, and red pepper flakes until everything is well combined. Cover and set aside for 20 to 30 minutes at room temperature, stirring periodically. Serve over rice that has been cooked.

Nutritional Information: Calories: 250 kcal, protein: 5 g, carbohydrates: 44 g, Fat: 6 g, Cholesterol: 0 mg, Fiber: 2 g

Grilled Veggie Subs

Preparation time: 5 minutes/**Cooking Time:** 20 minutes/**Total time:** 25 minutes

Servings: 4/**Difficulty Level:** Medium

Ingredients:

- 4 slices red onion
- 1/2 cup mushrooms, sliced
- 1/2 cup zucchini, sliced
- 3/4 cup eggplant, sliced
- 1 cup tomato, sliced
- 2 tablespoons olive oil
- 8 ounces Swiss cheese, sliced
- 8 slices focaccia bread or 4 rolls

Instructions

Preheat broiler. Brush onion, mushrooms, zucchini, eggplant, and tomato with oil. Grill or sauté until soft. Divide evenly between focaccia or rolls. Top each with a slice of Swiss cheese. Place under the broiler until cheese melts.

Nutritional Information: Calories: 192 kcal, protein: 17 g, carbohydrates: 9 g, Fat: 10 g, Cholesterol: 20 mg, Fiber: 2 g

Hawaiian Portobello Burgers

Preparation time: 15 minutes/**Cooking Time:** 20 minutes/**Total time:** 35 minutes

Servings: 2/**Difficulty Level:** Medium

Ingredients:

- 2 Portobello mushrooms, cleaned and stems removed
- 2 tablespoons Reduced-Sodium Teriyaki Sauce
- 2 slices pineapple
- 2 slices low fat Monterey jack cheese
- 2 lettuce leaves
- 2 slices tomato
- 2 hamburger buns
- 1 tablespoon low-fat mayonnaise

Instructions

Place mushrooms in a shallow dish. Spread teriyaki sauce over the mushrooms and marinate for 15 minutes. Grill the mushrooms and pineapple slices over low heat until tender. Add the cheese to the mushrooms and briefly grill to melt the cheese. Assemble burgers by placing 1 lettuce leaf and tomato slice on each bottom bun, then top with the mushrooms and pineapple. Spread each top bun with half of the mayonnaise.

Nutritional Information: Calories: 248 kcal, protein: 17 g, carbohydrates: 39 g, Fat: 6 g, Cholesterol: 9 mg, Fiber: 11 g

Roasted Vegetable Stuffed Pizza

Preparation time: 20 minutes/**Cooking Time:** 60 minutes/**Total time:** 1 hour 20 minutes/**Servings:** 6/**Difficulty Level:** Medium

Ingredients:

- 1 cup water
- 4 teaspoons olive oil
- 1 1/2 cups bread flour
- 1 1/2 cups whole wheat flour
- 1 1/2 teaspoons yeast
- 3 cups mushrooms, quartered
- 2 cups zucchini, sliced
- 1 cup onion, sliced
- 1 cup red bell pepper, sliced
- 1 cup green bell pepper, sliced
- 1 tablespoon olive oil
- 1 cup low sodium spaghetti sauce
- 3 ounces part-skim mozzarella, shredded

Instructions

Preheat oven to 450°F (230°C, or gas mark 8). Place the first 5 ingredients (through yeast) in a bread machine pan in the order specified by the manufacturer. Process on the dough cycle. Meanwhile, combine mushrooms, zucchini, onion, red and green bell peppers, and olive oil in a large baking pan. Bake vegetable mixture for 20 minutes, or until tender and browned on the edges. Stir in spaghetti sauce and set aside. Reduce oven heat to 350°F (180°C, or gas mark 4). Grease the bottom and sides of a 9-inch (23-cm) springform pan. When the dough is done, remove it from the bread machine, punch down, and rest for 10 minutes. Separate into two balls, with about three-quarters of the dough in the largest one. Roll the large bailout to a 16-inch (40-cm) circle. Place in the bottom and up the sides of the pan. Sprinkle half the cheese on the bottom. Place the vegetable mixture on the cheese, then sprinkle the remaining cheese. Roll the smaller ball to a 9-inch (23-cm) circle. Place over the mixture. Fold the edges of the bottom crust over the top and seal. Bake for 30 to 40 minutes, or until golden brown. Cool in pan 20 minutes, then remove sides and cut into six wedges.

Nutritional Information: Calories: 393 kcal, protein: 15 g, carbohydrates: 62 g, Fat: 11 g, Cholesterol: 9 mg, Fiber: 8 g

Vegetarian Lasagna

Preparation time: 15 minutes/**Cooking Time:** 1 hour 15 minutes/**Total time:** 1 hour 30 minutes7**Servings:** 12/**Difficulty Level:** Medium

Ingredients:

- 2 tablespoons olive oil
- 1 cup onion, chopped
- 6 cups low sodium spaghetti sauce
- 1 2 ounces frozen spinach, thawed and drained
- 15 ounces ricotta cheese
- 1/2 cup Parmesan, shredded
- 4 ounces part-skim mozzarella, shredded
- 2 tablespoons dried parsley
- 1/2 cup egg substitute
- 1 2 ounces lasagna noodles, cooked and drained

Instructions

Preheat oven to 350°F (180°C, or gas mark 4). In a large skillet, heat the olive oil over medium-high heat. Lightly sauté the onion in a skillet. Stir in spaghetti sauce. Mix the spinach, ricotta, Parmesan, mozzarella, parsley, and egg substitute in a large bowl. Spray a 9 x 13-inch (23 x 33-cm) baking pan with nonstick vegetable oil spray. Place a layer of tomato sauce in the bottom of the pan. Layer noodles, tomato sauce, and ricotta mixture in that order-making three layers of each. Add a layer of noodles and sauce to the top. Bake, covered with foil, for 60 to 75 minutes, or until bubbling and heated through. Remove the foil and bake 10 minutes longer.

Nutritional Information: Calories: 376 kcal, protein: 16 g, carbohydrates: 46 g, Fat: 15 g, Cholesterol: 21 mg, Fiber: 6 g

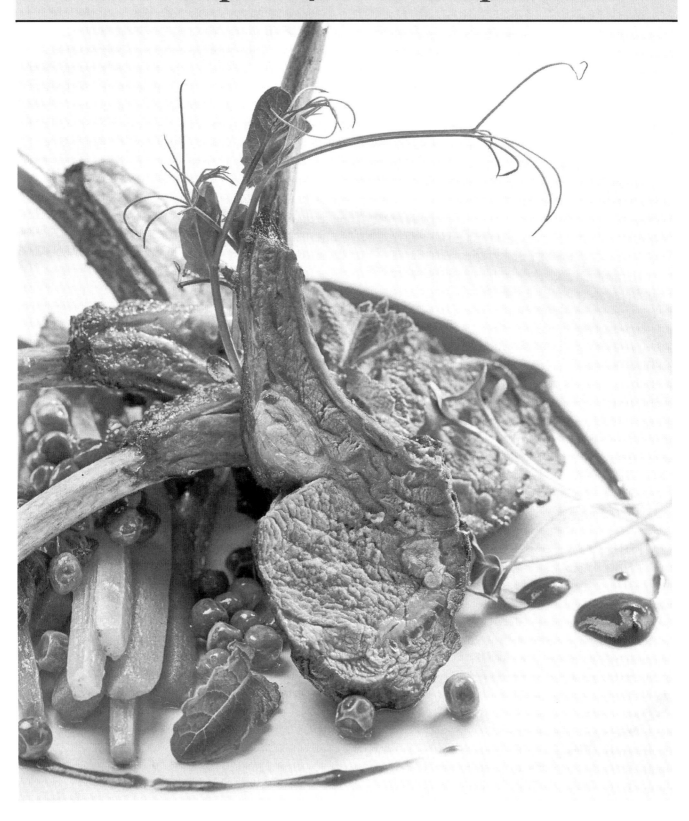

Flank Steak with Caramelized Onions

Preparation time: 10 minutes/**Cooking Time:** 30 minutes/**Total time:** 40 minutes

Servings: 4/**Difficulty Level:** Medium

Ingredients

- 2 large thinly sliced and halved lengthwise red onions,
- 1 tablespoon of butter
- 1/2 teaspoon of dried sage
- 1 green or red bell pepper; thin strips
- 11 -1/4 to 1 1/2 pounds, beef flank steak,
- 1/2 teaspoon of dried oregano
- 1 tablespoon of black pepper; freshly ground.
- 1/2 teaspoon of salt
- 1 15-ounce can black beans rinsed and drained, warmed.
- 4 7- to 8-inch warmed flour tortillas,

Instructions

In a large pan over medium heat, melt the butter. Cover and simmer onions in it, occasionally turning, until they are soft, for approximately 7 minutes. Add sage, bell pepper strips, and oregano. Cook, uncovered, over medium-high heat for 4 to 5 minutes, or until the peppers are crisp-tender and the onions are golden, stirring frequently. Preheat the grill pan to medium-high temperature. Trim the fat off the steak and score it on both sides with shallow diamond cuts at 1-inch intervals. Season with salt and pepper. Grill, rotating once, for 8 to 12 minutes for the medium-rare or 12 to 15 minutes for the medium. Thinly slice steak across the grain diagonally and cover it with onion mixture. Warm the tortillas and black beans are served on the side.

Nutritional Information:

Calories: 434 kcal, protein: 40 g, carbohydrates: 36 g, Fat: 15 g, Cholesterol: 37 mg, Fiber: 3.4 g

Juicy Burgers

Preparation time: 10 minutes/**Cooking Time:** 10 minutes/**Total time:** 20 minutes

Servings: 5/**Difficulty Level:** Easy

Ingredients

- 1 cup low sodium beef broth
- 2 slices white bread, torn into pieces
- 1 1/2 pounds' extra-lean ground beef (93% lean)
- 2 tablespoons egg substitute
- 1/2 teaspoon black pepper

Instructions

Microwave broth in a glass bowl for 30 seconds. Add bread pieces and combine with your hands. Combine broth mixture and remaining ingredients. Shape into 5 patties. Grill patties over medium-high heat for 6 to 8 minutes on each side or to desired doneness.

Nutritional Information: Calories: 328 kcal, protein: 27 g, carbohydrates: 0 g, Fat: 9 g, Cholesterol: 94 mg, Fiber: 0 g

Steak & Vegetables with Chimichurri Sauce

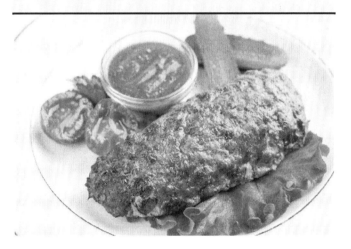

Preparation time: 20 minutes/**Cooking Time:** 40 minutes/**Total time:** 60 minutes

Servings: 4/**Difficulty Level:** Medium

Ingredients

Steak & Vegetables

- ½ teaspoon of chili powder
- 1 pound of top sirloin beef steak; boneless, 1 inch thick
- ¼ teaspoon of salt

- 1 small red onion, 1/2-inch-thick slices
- 2 cups of cherry tomatoes or grape tomatoes
- Nonstick cooking spray
- 2 medium-trimmed zucchini or yellow summer squash halved lengthwise.

Chimichurri Sauce

- ½ cup of fresh cilantro; lightly packed
- 1 cup of fresh, lightly packed flat-leaf parsley
- ¼ cup of white wine vinegar
- 1 tablespoon of olive oil
- 2 tablespoons of water
- ¼ teaspoon of salt
- 6 minced cloves of garlic,
- ¼ teaspoon of crushed red pepper (Optional)
- ¼ teaspoon of ground black pepper

Instructions

Trim the fat off the steak. Use a knife to cut the meat into four equal pieces. Season the steak pieces with 1/8 teaspoon of salt and chili powder. Using four 6- to 8-inch skewers, thread tomatoes onto the skewers. Lightly brush the zucchini, tomatoes, and red onion slices on both sides with nonstick spray. Sprinkle the remaining 1/8 tsp of salt into the veggies.

Place tomato skewers, steak, and vegetable slices on the uncovered grill rack directly over medium embers using a charcoal grill. Grill the steak until it reaches your preferred level of doneness, flipping once halfway through. Allow it 14 to 18 minutes for the medium-rare doneness (145 degrees Fahrenheit) or 18 to 22 minutes for the medium doneness (145 degrees Fahrenheit) to (160 degrees F). Grill onion slices and zucchini for 10 to 12 minutes, turning periodically, until soft and faintly browned in spots. Grill the tomatoes for 4 to 6 minutes, rotating once, or until softened and faintly browned. (Preheat the grill if using a gas grill.) Reduce to a medium heat setting. Place the tomato skewers, steak, and vegetable slices on the grill rack and cook them over high heat. Cover and cook as directed above).

Chimichurri Sauce Preparation: In a blender or food processor, combine cilantro, parsley, vinegar, olive oil, water, garlic, ground black pepper, salt, and, if preferred, crushed red pepper. Cover and mix or pulse several times on/off until chopped but not pureed. Using four serving dishes, divide the sliced meat. Grilled tomatoes, Chimichurri sauce, and veggie pieces are served on the side.

Nutritional Information: Calories: 245 kcal, protein: 28.3 g, carbohydrates: 13.1 g, Fat: 8.6 g, Cholesterol: 47.6 mg, Fiber: 3.7 g

Beef Noodle Soup

Preparation time: 5 minutes/**Cooking Time:** 25 minutes/**Total time:** 30 minutes

Servings: 4/**Difficulty Level:** Medium

Ingredients:

- 3 small Baby Bok Choy; halved
- 1 tsp of Oil
- 2 stalks of Spring Onions; diced
- 6 cups of Beef Broth; Low Sodium
- 2 tbsp. of Soy Sauce; Reduced Sodium
- 1/2 tsp of Fresh Ginger Root; grated
- 2 1/2 cup of Zucchini
- 1/4 cup of Thai Basil, shredded
- 1 1/4 lbs. Lean Beef; sliced
- 1/4 tsp of Red Pepper Crushed Flakes
- 1 tsp of Sesame Oil
- 1/4 tsp of Black Pepper

Instructions

Cook the spring onions and Baby Bok Choy in a wok or pan with oil. Combine soy sauce, broth, and ginger in a large soup pot. Bring to a low simmer after covering it.

Add the steak strips to the soup after slicing it as thinly as possible. Simmer the soup to a moderate boil, then reduce to low heat, cover, and cook until the meat is fully cooked. Remove the soup from the heat and stir in the zucchini noodles. Add sesame oil, black pepper, basil, and crushed red pepper flakes. Serve hot with an equal quantity of soup in each dish.

Nutritional Information: Calories: 361 kcal, protein: 15.4 g, carbohydrates: 32.1 g, Fat: 19 g, Cholesterol: 12.2 mg, Fiber: 4.4 g

BBQ Pulled Pork with Greek Yogurt Slaw

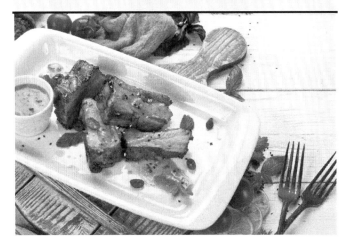

Preparation time: 10 minutes/**Cooking Time:** 1 hour /**Total time:** 1 hour 10 minutes

Servings: 4/**Difficulty Level:** Medium

Ingredients:

- 3 cups of Green Cabbage; shredded
- 1/2 cup of Non-Fat Plain Greek Yogurt
- 3 cups of Red Cabbage; shredded
- 1 (12oz.) can of Diet Root Beer
- 2 tsp of Lemon Juice
- 1 tbsp. of Apple Cider Vinegar
- 1/4 tsp of Celery Salt
- 1 tsp of Dijon Mustard
- 1 can of Light Cooking Spray
- 1 1/2 lbs. Pork Tenderloin; halved
- 1 pinch Stevia
- 4 sachets of Buttermilk Cheddar Herb Biscuit
- 1/2 cup of BBQ Sauce; Sugar-Free

Instructions

Cooking spray is used to coat the interior of the Instant Pot. On a high sauté ' setting, brown the pork chunks on all sides, approximately 3 minutes on each side.

Close the pressure valve after adding the diet root beer. Set the timer for 60 minutes on high. Allow for natural pressure release before opening. Prepare the slaw in the meanwhile. Combine cabbage, yogurt, apple cider vinegar, lemon juice, Dijon mustard, salt, and stevia in a medium-sized mixing bowl.

Remove the pork from the Instant Pot and shred it in a bowl. Toss in the barbecue sauce and mix well. Bake

Herb Biscuits according to package instructions, if desired. Serve the slaw and shredded pork on top of biscuits or without baked biscuits.

Nutritional Information: Calories: 108 kcal, protein: 5.8 g, carbohydrates: 14 g, Fat: 2.5 g, Cholesterol: 39.9 mg, Fiber: 3.5 g

Mexican Stuffed Peppers with Corn and Black Beans

Preparation time: 10 minutes/**Cooking Time:** 30 minutes/**Total time:** 40 minutes
Servings: 6/**Difficulty Level:** Medium
Ingredients:

- 6 bell peppers; any color
- 1 tablespoon of olive oil
- 1 chopped yellow onion,
- 2 minced cloves of garlic,
- 1 pound of lean ground beef
- 1 tablespoon of chili powder
- 1 1/2 teaspoons of ground cumin
- 1 (4-ounce) can have diced green chiles
- 1 1/2 cups of cooked white rice
- 2 medium diced tomatoes,
- 1 (15-ounce) can have drained and rinsed black beans,
- 1 cup of defrosted frozen corn,
- 1/2 cup of shredded Cheddar cheese or Mexican-blend
- Optional toppings: Chopped fresh cilantro or green onions.

Instructions

Preheat the oven to 350 degrees Fahrenheit. A big pot of water is brought to a boil. Slice the peppers in half vertically through the center of the stem and to the bottom. Remove the membranes as well as the seeds.

For 3–4 minutes, until the peppers are somewhat softened, parboil them in a saucepan of water. Drain the peppers and arrange them cut side up in a wide baking dish. Warm the oil in a wide skillet over medium heat. Sauté for 4 minutes, or until the onion is transparent. Cook for another minute after adding the garlic.

Cook for 5 minutes, or until the ground beef is brown, frequently stirring to break up the meat. Chili powder, green chiles, cooked rice, black beans, tomatoes, cumin, and maize are added. Season with pepper and salt to taste. Fill the peppers halfway with the ground beef rice mixture and top with cheese. Bake for 15-20 minutes, or until the peppers are soft and the cheese has melted. If using, garnish with cilantro or green onions and serve warm.

Nutritional Information: Calories: 357 kcal, protein: 26 g, carbohydrates: 46 g, Fat: 7 g, Cholesterol: 46 mg, Fiber: 3 g

Meatloaf

Preparation time: 10 minutes/**Cooking Time:** 1-1 ½ hour/**Total time:** 1 hour 40 minutes/**Servings:** 6/**Difficulty Level:** Medium

Ingredients:

- 1 1/2 pounds extra-lean ground beef (93% lean)
- 1 cup breadcrumbs
- 1 onion, finely chopped
- 1/4 cup egg substitute
- 1/4 teaspoon black pepper
- 8 ounces no-salt-added tomato sauce, divided
- 1/2 cup water
- 2 teaspoons Worcestershire sauce
- 3 tablespoons vinegar
- 2 tablespoons mustard
- 3 tablespoons brown sugar

Instructions

Preheat oven to 350°F (180°C, or gas mark 4). Mix beef, breadcrumbs, onion, egg substitute, pepper, and half the tomato sauce. Form into one large loaf or two small ones; mix remaining tomato sauce and remaining ingredients together; pour over loaves. Bake for 1 to 1 1/2 hours.

Nutritional Information: Calories: 393 kcal, protein: 26 g, carbohydrates: 23 g, Fat: 9 g, Cholesterol: 78 mg, Fiber: 1 g

Oaxacan Tacos

Preparation time: 10 minutes/**Cooking Time:** 15 minutes/**Total time:** 25 minutes

Servings: 9/**Difficulty Level:** Medium

Ingredients

- ground black pepper and salt to taste
- 2 pounds of top sirloin steak, thin strips
- 4 limes, wedges
- ¼ cup of vegetable oil
- 1 diced onion,
- 18 corn tortillas; (6 inches)
- 1 bunch of fresh cilantro; chopped,
- 4 fresh seeded and chopped jalapeno peppers,

Instructions

In a large skillet, heat the oil over medium-high heat. Put meat in the tit and cook for 5 minutes in a hot pan until the steak is browned on the outer side and is cooked through. Sprinkle salt & pepper to taste. Place on a platter to keep warm. In the same skillet, heat the oil. Put the tortilla in the heated oil and cook until lightly browned and pliable, flipping once. Continue with the remaining tortillas. On a platter, arrange tortillas and top with steak, jalapeño, onion, and cilantro. Lime juice should be squeezed over the top.

Nutritional Information: Calories: 379 kcal, protein: 20.3 g, carbohydrates: 28.1 g, Fat: 21.4 g, Cholesterol: 58.5 mg, Fiber: 1 g

Beef and Broccoli Teriyaki Noodle Bowls

Preparation time: 45 minutes/**Cooking Time:** 20 minutes/**Total time:** 1 hour 10 minutes/**Servings:** 4/**Difficulty Level:** Medium

Ingredients:

- 1 thinly sliced onion
- 1 1/4 teaspoon of dried ginger
- 4 ounces of thin rice noodles
- 1/4 cup of tamari sauce
- 3 cups of broccoli florets
- 1 ½ pound of skirt steak; thinly sliced against the grain.
- 1/4 teaspoon of red pepper flakes
- 3/4 cup of teriyaki sauce; gluten-free

Instructions:

Fill a large microwave-safe bowl halfway with water and microwave for 3 minutes, or until the water is extremely hot. Remove the water from the microwave and place noodles in the water. Allow 45 minutes for soaking.

Begin preparing the meat once the noodles have soaked for 30 minutes:

Over medium heat, sauté the cut onions and meat in a large pan. Cook until done, stirring often. Whisk the gluten-free teriyaki sauce, ginger, tamari sauce, and red pepper flakes in a small mixing bowl. Fill the skillet with the sauce. Stir everything together well. In the same skillet, add the broccoli.

Microwave the noodles for 2-3 minutes in water. Drain. Combine the meat, noodles, broccoli, and sauce in a pan. Toss to coat. Serve right away.

Nutritional Information: Calories: 456 kcal, protein: 44 g, carbohydrates: 40 g, Fat: 13 g, Cholesterol: 85 mg, Fiber: 2 g

Mexican Skillet Meal

Preparation time: 5 minutes/**Cooking Time:** 30 minutes/**Total time:** 35 minutes

Servings: 5/**Difficulty Level:** Medium

Ingredients:

- 1-pound extra-lean ground beef (93% lean)
- 1/2 cup onion, chopped
- 1/4 cup green bell peppers, chopped
- 1/4 cup red bell pepper, chopped
- 1/2 teaspoon minced garlic
- 1 1/2 cups rice
- 3 cups water
- 2 teaspoons low sodium beef bouillon
- 2 cups canned no-salt-added tomatoes
- 1 tablespoon chili powder
- 1/2 teaspoon cumin
- 1/4 teaspoon dried oregano
- 1 2 ounces frozen corn, thawed

Instructions:

Sauté beef, onion, green and red bell peppers, and garlic in a large skillet until beef is browned and vegetables are tender. Add rice and sauté 2 minutes longer. Stir in the remaining ingredients. Bring to boil. Reduce heat, cover, and simmer for 20 minutes, or until rice is tender and liquid is absorbed.

Nutritional Information: Calories: 357 kcal, protein: 22 g, carbohydrates: 33 g, Fat: 7 g, Cholesterol: 63 mg, Fiber: 4 g

Bistecca alla Fiorentina Steak

Preparation time: 1 hour 20 minutes /**Cooking Time:** 20 minutes/**Total time:** 1 hour 40 minutes/**Servings:** 6/**Difficulty Level:** Medium

Ingredients

- 1 prime porterhouse steak (2- 1/2 pound)
- 4 sprigs of chopped fresh rosemary,
- 3 tablespoons of Tuscan olive oil
- 6 lemon wedges
- Grey moist, pepper, and sea salt to taste, freshly cracked.

Instructions

This dish is also known as Tuscan Peter house steak.

Hardwood charcoal can be used to start an outdoor grill. Spread chopped rosemary on all sides of steak, place on a platter, and leave aside to marinate for 1 hour at room temperature. Arrange for maximum heat when the coals are white and blazing.

Brush or massage olive oil over the steak, then season with sea salt & pepper to taste. Place steak on the grill and cook for 5 to 10 mins, depending on the thickness of the meat, until dark golden brown (not burned) crust develops. Cook for another 5 to 10 mins, or until golden brown on the opposite side. Place the steak on a plate and set it aside to sit for 10 mins.

Remove the 2 pieces off the bone and put them on the serving plate. Trim any excess fat from round steak (tenderloin) before slicing it into 6 equal pieces and fanning them out on one side of the bone. Slice the rectangular steak (loin) into 1/4-inch pieces at an angle to the grain. On the other side of the bone, fan out. Finish with lemon wedges and a sprinkling of sea salt on top of the dish.

Nutritional Information: Calories: 346 kcal, protein: 18.2 g, carbohydrates: 1.5 g, Fat: 29.6 g, Cholesterol: 62.8 mg, Fiber: 3 g

Tailgate Chili

Preparation time: 5 minutes /**Cooking Time:** 35 minutes/**Total time:** 40 minutes

Servings: 4/**Difficulty Level:** Medium

Ingredients

- 1 medium chopped onion
- 1 lb. ground beef; 95% lean
- 1 medium chopped jalapeño
- 1 medium green chopped bell pepper
- 1 Tbsp. of chili powder
- 4 cloves of fresh garlic; minced, OR 2 tsp. of jarred minced garlic.
- 1/2 tsp. of ground coriander
- 1 Tbsp. of ground cumin
- 15.5 oz. Canned, low-sodium, or no-salt-added pinto/kidney beans, rinsed and drained.
- 3/4 cup of jarred salsa (low sodium)
- 14.5 oz. of canned, low-sodium or no-salt-added, diced tomatoes (undrained)

Instructions

Use a cooking spray to coat a big pot. Add and cook beef for 5-7 minutes over medium-high heat, frequently stirring to break up the meat. Drain excess fat in a strainer by rinsing with water. Return the meat into the pot. Cook for 5 minutes, stirring periodically, after adding the chili powder, garlic, bell pepper, and cumin. Bring the remaining ingredients to a boil. Reduce the heat to a low, cover, and cook for 20 minutes. If desired, serve with fat-free sour cream, low-fat grated cheese, sliced avocado, chopped green onions, or trimmed cilantro.

Nutritional Information: Calories: 297 kcal, protein: 31 g, carbohydrates: 29 g, Fat: 6 g, Cholesterol: 62 mg, Fiber: 7 g

London Broil

Preparation time: 5 minutes /**Cooking Time:** 15 minutes/**Total time:** 20 minutes

Servings: 5/**Difficulty Level:** Medium

Ingredients

- 1/4 cup olive oil

- 1 teaspoon cider vinegar
- 1/4 teaspoon minced garlic
- 1/4 teaspoon freshly ground black pepper
- 1 1/2 pounds beef round steak

Instructions

Score steak on both sides. Combine oil, vinegar, garlic, and pepper in a resalable plastic bag. Add steak and marinate for several hours, turning occasionally. Preheat broiler. Remove steak from marinade and broil 3 inches (7.5 cm) from heat for 4 to 5 minutes. Turn and broil 4 to 5 minutes longer, or until medium-rare. Carve in thin slices against the grain.

Nutritional Information: Calories: 367 kcal, protein: 49 g, carbohydrates: 0 g, Fat: 18 g, Cholesterol: 122 mg, Fiber: 0 g

Mojo Flat Iron Steak

Preparation time: 40 minutes /**Cooking Time:** 20 minutes/**Total time:** 1 hour

Servings: 4/**Difficulty Level:** Medium

Ingredients

- 1 teaspoon of chili powder
- 2 teaspoons of brown sugar
- 1 (1-pound) trimmed flat iron steak,
- ¼ cup of fresh orange juice
- 2 teaspoons of grated orange rind
- ¼ teaspoon of chipotle chile powder; ground
- 2 minced garlic cloves,
- 1 teaspoon of kosher salt; divided.
- Cooking spray
- 2 teaspoons of grated lime rind
- 1 cup of peeled, seeded cucumber; finely chopped.
- 2 tablespoons of olive oil; extra-virgin, divided.
- 3 tablespoons of fresh lime juice, divided.
- 1 cup of red bell pepper; finely chopped.
- 3 tablespoons of red onion; finely chopped.
- ¼ cup of fresh orange juice
- 1 seeded and finely chopped jalapeño pepper,
- 2 tablespoons of chopped fresh cilantro.

Instructions

In a mixing bowl, whisk the orange juice, orange rind, lime rind, 1 tablespoon oil, 2 tablespoons lime juice, cloves, brown sugar, chili powder, and chipotle chile powder. Add the steak and turn to cover it with the sauce. Allow it to sit at room temperature for 30 minutes, rotating periodically.

Preheat a grill pan to high. Spray the pan with nonstick cooking spray. Remove the meat from the marinade and discard the marinade. Using 1/2 teaspoon of salt, season the meat. Add the steak to the pan and cook it for 5 minutes on each side for medium-rare or until desired doneness is reached. Place the steak on a chopping board and let it rest for 5 minutes. Using a sharp knife, cut steak across the grain. In a mixing dish, combine the remaining 1 tablespoon oil, 1/2 teaspoon salt, 1 tablespoon of lime juice, and the other ingredients. Serve alongside a steak.

Nutritional Information: Calories: 216 kcal, protein: 24 g, carbohydrates: 6 g, Fat: 11.1 g, Cholesterol: 81 mg, Fiber: 1 g

Beef Fajita

Preparation time: 10 minutes /**Cooking Time:** 15-20 minutes/**Total time:** 30 minutes/**Servings:** 4/**Difficulty Level:** Medium

Ingredients:

- ¼ Red pepper; thinly sliced.
- 1 Corn tortilla
- ¼ Red onion; thinly sliced.
- Beef 60 g; cut it into pieces.
- ¼ Green pepper; thinly sliced.
- 1 tsp of Plain yogurt
- 1 tbsp of Cilantro; Chopped.
- ½ tsp of Olive oil
- ¼ tsp of Chili powder

Instructions

Heat the oil in a skillet before adding the onion and peppers. After adding the beef, cook for another 3 minutes or until beef is cooked through. Combine the chili powder and yogurt in a small bowl and distribute them over the tortilla. Place all cooked items on the tortilla, along with the cilantro, and serve.

Nutritional Information: Calories: 225 kcal, protein: 14.2 g, carbohydrates: 12.9 g, Fat: 11 g, Cholesterol: 35 mg, Fiber: 2.9 g

Bulgogi Ground Beef

Preparation time: 5 minutes /**Cooking Time:** 15-20 minutes/**Total time:** 25 minutes

Servings: 4/**Difficulty Level:** Medium

Ingredients:

- 1/2 teaspoon of red pepper flakes; crushed.
- 1/4 cup of coconut sugar
- 3 minced cloves of garlic,
- 1/4 cup of organic tamari (low sodium gluten-free soy sauce)
- 2 teaspoons of sesame oil
- 1 tablespoon of grated ginger
- Optional toppings: Sesame seeds, sliced green onions, and sliced red chiles.
- 1 pound of lean ground beef

Instructions

Whisk the coconut sugar, tamari, and red pepper flakes in a small bowl. Put it aside. Heat sesame oil in a large pan over medium heat. Add ginger and garlic. Sauté for 1 minute, or until they are aromatic. Add the beef and cook it for approximately 5 minutes, or until the ground beef is fully browned, frequently stirring to break up the meat. Stir in the tamari mixture until everything is well blended. Allow mixture to boil for 2 minutes, or until well heated. Garnish with desired toppings and serve it warm over the cooked rice.

Nutritional Information: Calories: 220 kcal, protein: 26 g, carbohydrates: 11 g, Fat: 8 g, Cholesterol: 70 mg, Fiber: 3 g

Shredded Beef Tacos

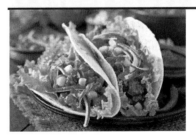

Preparation time: 4 hours 30 minutes /**Cooking Time:** 2 ½ hours/**Total time:** 7 hours/**Servings:** 4/**Difficulty Level:** Medium

Ingredients:

- 2 tablespoons of vinegar

- ¼ cup of vegetable oil
- 1 ½ teaspoon of ground cumin
- 2 tablespoons of lime juice
- 3 minced cloves of garlic,
- 1 ½ teaspoon of chili powder
- 1 ½ pound of beef chuck roast; trim it, 1-inch-thick slices
- salt to taste
- 1 cup of beef stock

Instructions

Combine the vinegar, vegetable oil, lime juice, chili powder, cumin, and garlic; pour it into a resalable plastic bag. Add the sliced beef to the bag, cover it with the marinade, press out any air, and close it. Marinate for 4 hours or overnight in the refrigerator.

Preheat the oven to 350 degrees Fahrenheit (175 degrees C). Place the meat with the lime juice marinade in a large baking dish. Cover the baking dish with aluminum foil after adding the beef stock. Bake it for 2 1/2 hours in a preheated oven until the meat is extremely tender. Allow 20 minutes for the meat to come to room temperature. Allow 10 minutes for the meat to rest before shredding with two forks. Before serving, drain and discard approximately 80% of the liquid from the meat.

Nutritional Information: Calories: 399 kcal, protein: 21.2 g, carbohydrates: 3.1 g, Fat: 33.3 g, Cholesterol: 77.2 mg, Fiber: 4 g

Beef Tenderloin and Balsamic Tomatoes

Preparation time: 5 minutes /**Cooking Time:** 20 minutes/**Total time:** 25 minutes

Servings: 2/**Difficulty Level:** Medium

Ingredients:

- ⅓ cup of seeded tomato; coarsely chopped,
- ½ cup of balsamic vinegar
- 2 teaspoons of olive oil
- 1 teaspoon of snipped fresh thyme
- 2 (about 8 ounces) beef tenderloin steaks, 3/4 inch thick

Instructions

Bring vinegar to a boil in a small saucepan. Reduce heat to low and cook, uncovered, for 5 minutes, or until liquid is reduced to a 1/4 cup. Tomatoes are stirred into the hot vinegar reduction.

Trim the fat from the steaks in the meanwhile. Season to taste with pepper and salt. Warm the oil in a wide skillet over medium-high heat. Reduce the heat to medium-low and add the steaks. Cook until done to your liking, flipping once. For the medium-rare (145°F) to the medium (160°F), allow 7 to 9 minutes. Pour the vinegar reduction over the steaks to serve. Thyme is sprinkled on top.

Nutritional Information: Calories: 275 kcal, protein: 26 g, carbohydrates: 12 g, Fat: 12 g, Cholesterol: 76 mg, Fiber: 10 g

Spaghetti Squash Casserole with ground beef

Preparation time: 10 minutes /**Cooking Time:** 1 hour 20 minutes/**Total time:** 1 hour 30 minutes/**Servings:** 8/**Difficulty Level:** Medium

Ingredients:

- Non-stick cooking spray
- 2 medium spaghetti squash
- 1-pound supreme lean ground beef
- 2 teaspoons minced garlic
- 1 (8-ounce) can tomato sauce
- 1 large onion minced.
- 1 (10-ounce) can diced tomatoes
- 1 teaspoon of dried basil
- 1 teaspoon of dried oregano
- 1 cup shredded mozzarella cheese
- ½ cup shredded Parmigiano-Reggiano cheese

Instructions:

Preheat the oven to 350 degrees F. Coat a baking sheet with the cooking spray. Halve the spaghetti squash, remove, discard the stem, pulp, and seeds and place halves cut-side down on the baking sheet. Bake for about 35 minutes or until tender. While the squash bakes, spray a large skillet with the cooking spray, and over medium heat, place it. Add ground beef, onion, and garlic and sauté for about 10 minutes or until the beef is no longer pink and the onion is tender. Add the tomato sauce, diced tomatoes, basil, oregano, and stir to combine well. Remove the pan from heat and set it aside. When the spaghetti squash is cool enough to handle carefully, use a fork, pull the flesh from the outer skin, and make spaghetti. Set aside in a bowl. In a 9 by 13-inch baking dish, layer one-third of the meat and tomato mixture in the bottom of the dish. Evenly spread half of the squash over the meat layer. Assemble another layer in the same pattern over it. Last, sprinkle cheese over the top. Cover with aluminum foil and bake for 30 minutes. Remove the foil and bake for more than 10 minutes or until cheese brown. Serve warm.

Nutritional Information: Calories: 229 kcal, protein: 20 g, carbohydrates: 16 g, Fat: 10 g, Cholesterol: 56 mg, Fiber: 3 g

Sloppy Joes

Preparation time: 10 minutes /**Cooking Time:** 30 minutes/**Total time:** 40 minutes

Servings: 8/**Difficulty Level:** Medium

Ingredients:

- non-stick cooking spray
- 1 ½ pound supreme lean ground beef
- 1 cup chopped onion.
- 1 cup chopped celery.
- 1 (8-ounce) can tomato sauce
- 1/3 cup catsup (free of high fructose)
- 2 tablespoons white vinegar
- 2 tablespoons Worcestershire sauce
- 2 tablespoons Dijon mustard
- 1 tablespoon brown sugar

Instructions:

Spray a large skillet with the cooking spray and place it over medium heat. Add the beef and brown until it is no longer pink, about 10 minutes. Drain off any grease. Mix in the onion and celery and cook for 2 to 3 minutes. Stir in the tomato sauce, catsup, vinegar, Worcestershire sauce, mustard, and brown sugar. Bring the liquid to a simmer and reduce the heat to low. Cook for 15 minutes or until the sauce has thickened. Spoon about ¾ cup of the sloppy joe mixture onto each plate and serve.

Nutritional Information: Calories: 269 kcal, protein: 24 g, carbohydrates: 32 g, Fat: 5 g, Cholesterol: 56.7 mg, Fiber: 6 g

Italian Beef Roast

Preparation time: 10 minutes /**Cooking Time:** 2 hours 40 minutes/**Total time:** 2 hours 50 minutes/**Servings:** 10/**Difficulty Level:** Medium

Ingredients:

- 1/2 cup dry red wine
- 2 tablespoons Italian seasoning
- 4 pounds beef round tip roast
- 1 cup low sodium spaghetti sauce
- 1 cup onion, sliced
- 1 cup celery, sliced
- 1 cup mushrooms, sliced
- 1/2 cup fat-free sour cream
- 1/4 cup water
- 1/4 cup flour

Instructions:
Combine wine and Italian seasoning. Marinate roast in the mixture overnight. In a Dutch oven, combine marinade and spaghetti sauce. Add roast. Cover and simmer for 1 1/2 hours. Add onion, celery, and mushrooms, cover, and simmer for 1 hour, or until meat is tender. Remove roast and vegetables. Skim fat off pan juices and return 2 cups (470 ml) liquid to pan. Combine sour cream and water. Stir in flour. Stir sour cream mixture into the pan juices and simmer until thickened. Serve sauce with meat.

Nutritional Information: Calories: 298 kcal, protein: 40 g, carbohydrates: 10 g, Fat: 7 g, Cholesterol: 101 mg, Fiber: 2 g

Meat and Mushrooms Bowl

Preparation time: 10 minutes /**Cooking Time:** 25 minutes/**Total time:** 35 minutes

Servings: 2/**Difficulty Level:** Easy

Ingredients:

- 6 oz pork sirloin, sliced
- 1 cup cremini mushrooms, sliced
- 1 tablespoon olive oil
- 1 teaspoon dried dill
- 1 teaspoon ground black pepper
- ½ cup low-fat yogurt

Instructions:

Roast sliced meat in the skillet for 5 minutes. Then stir it well and add dried dill, ground black pepper, and mushrooms. Cook the ingredients for 10 minutes on medium heat. After this, add yogurt and stir the ingredients well. Close the lid and cook the meal for 10 minutes more. Transfer the cooked meal to the serving bowls.

Nutritional Information: Calories: 269 kcal, protein: 22.1 g, carbohydrates: 6.8 g, Fat: 16.2 g, Cholesterol: 57 mg, Fiber: 0.6 g

Sauerbraten

Preparation time: 10 minutes plus marination time/**Cooking Time:** 2 hours 40 minutes/**Total time:** 2 hours 50 minutes/**Servings:** 10/**Difficulty Level:** Easy

Ingredients:

For Marinade:

- 2 1/2 cups water
- 1 1/2 cups red wine vinegar
- 1 tablespoon sugar
- 1/4 teaspoon ground ginger
- 1 2 whole cloves
- 6 bay leaves
- 2 cups onion, sliced

For Meat

- 4 pounds beef round roast
- 2 tablespoons olive oil
- 1/2 cup carrot, finely chopped
- 1/2 cup celery, finely chopped
- 1/2 cup onion, finely chopped
- 1 cup gingersnaps, crushed
- 2/3 cup water

Instructions:

To make the marinade: Combine the marinade ingredients in a large bowl. Add roast. Cover and refrigerate for 1 1/2 to 2 days, turning occasionally. Remove meat and wipe dry. Strain and reserve marinade liquid.

To make the meat: In a Dutch oven, brown meat in oil on all sides. Add reserved marinade, carrots, celery, and chopped onion. Cover and simmer until meat is tender, 2 to 2 1/2 hours. Remove meat to a platter and slice thinly. Reserve 2 cups of cooking liquid in the pot. Add gingersnaps and water. Cook and stir until thickened. Serve sauce with meat.

Nutritional Information: Calories: 323 kcal, protein: 41 g, carbohydrates: 12 g, Fat: 10 g, Cholesterol: 91 mg, Fiber: 1 g

Beef Kabobs

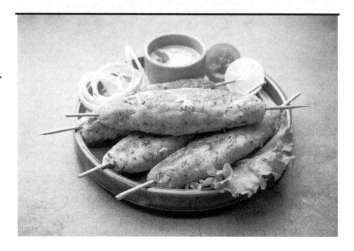

Preparation time: 10 minutes/**Cooking Time:** 30minutes/**Total time:** 40 minutes

Servings: 4/**Difficulty Level:** Easy

Ingredients:

- 1/4 cup olive oil
- 1/3 cup Reduced-Sodium Soy Sauce
- 1/4 cup lemon juice
- 2 tablespoons Worcestershire sauce
- 1/2 teaspoon minced garlic
- 1 teaspoon coarsely ground black pepper
- 1-pound beef round steak, cut in 1 -inch (2.5-cm) cubes
- 2 cups mushrooms

Instructions:

Mix all ingredients except beef and mushrooms. Add beef cubes. Cover and refrigerate overnight, turning meat occasionally. Thread meat and mushrooms on skewers. Grill over a fire to the desired doneness, turning often.

Nutritional Information: Calories: 380 kcal, protein: 42 g, carbohydrates: 135 g, Fat: 19 g, Cholesterol: 102 mg, Fiber: 1 g

Peasant Soup

Preparation time: 10 minutes/**Cooking Time:** 30 minutes/**Total time:** 40 minutes

Servings: 6/**Difficulty Level:** Easy

Ingredients:

- 1-pound leftover roast beef, chopped
- 2 cups low sodium beef broth
- 1 cup canned no-salt-added tomatoes
- 1-pound frozen mixed vegetables, thawed
- 1 cup cabbage, shredded
- 1/2 cup turnips, cubed

Instructions:

Combine all ingredients in a large Dutch oven. Simmer until vegetables are tender.

Nutritional Information: Calories: 198 kcal, protein: 25 g, carbohydrates: 13 g, Fat: 5 g, Cholesterol: 67 mg, Fiber: 4 g

Oven Swiss Steak

Preparation time: 10 minutes/**Cooking Time:** 2 hours/**Total time:** 2 hours 10 minutes/**Servings:** 6/**Difficulty Level:** Medium

Ingredients:

- 1 1/2 pounds beef round steak
- 1/4 cup flour
- 2 tablespoons olive oil
- 2 cups canned no-salt-added tomatoes
- 1/2 cup celery, finely chopped
- 1/2 cup carrot, finely chopped
- 1 tablespoon Worcestershire sauce

Instructions:

Preheat oven to 350°F (180°C, or gas mark 4). Cut meat into serving-sized pieces. Dredge in flour. Heat oil in a heavy skillet. Brown meat on both sides in oil. Transfer meat to a glass baking dish. Blend any remaining flour into pan drippings. Stir in the remaining ingredients. Cook and stir until thickened and bubbly. Pour over meat. Bake, covered, for 1 1/2 hours, or until tender.

Nutritional Information: Calories: 306 kcal, protein: 42 g, carbohydrates: 9 g, Fat: 10 g, Cholesterol: 102 mg, Fiber: 3 g

Enchilada Bake

Preparation time: 10 minutes/**Cooking Time:** 35 minutes/**Total time:** 45 minutes

Servings: 6/**Difficulty Level:** Medium

Ingredients:

- 1-pound extra-lean ground beef (93% lean)
- 1/4 cup onion, chopped
- 1 cup egg substitute
- 8 ounces no-salt-added tomato sauce
- 2/3 cup fat-free evaporated milk
- 2 tablespoons taco seasoning
- 1/4 cup ripe olives, sliced
- 1 cup corn chips
- 3/4 cup low-fat cheddar cheese, shredded

Instructions:

Preheat oven to 350°F (180°C, or gas mark 4). In a skillet, cook beef and onion until meat is brown and onion is soft. Drain. Spread in the bottom of a 9-inch (23-cm) square baking dish that has been coated with nonstick vegetable oil spray. Beat together egg substitute, tomato sauce, milk, and taco seasoning. Pour over meat. Sprinkle with olives. Top with corn chips. Bake for 25 minutes, or until set in the center. Sprinkle cheese on top and return to oven just until cheese melts, about 3 minutes.

Nutritional Information: Calories: 339 kcal, protein: 27 g, carbohydrates: 14 g, Fat: 11 g, Cholesterol: 57 mg, Fiber: 1 g

Chili Casserole

Preparation time: 10 minutes/**Cooking Time:** 30 minutes/**Total time:** 40 minutes

Servings: 4/**Difficulty Level:** Medium

Ingredients:

- 1-pound extra-lean ground beef (93% lean)
- 1/2 cup onion, chopped
- 1/2 cup red bell pepper, chopped
- 2 cups no-salt-added kidney beans

- 2 cups tomatoes, chopped and drained
- 1 cup frozen corn
- 1 tablespoon chili powder
- 1 teaspoon cumin
- 1/2 teaspoon garlic powder
- 1/2 cup flour
- 1/2 cup yellow cornmeal
- 2 tablespoons sugar
- 1 1/2 teaspoons baking powder
- 1 cup skim milk
- 1/4 cup egg substitute, or 1 egg
- 1 tablespoon olive oil

Instructions:

Preheat oven to 425°F (220°C, or gas mark 7). Brown beef with onions and red bell pepper until beef is no longer pink. Add beans, tomatoes, corn, chili powder, cumin, and garlic powder and simmer for 5 minutes. Stir together flour, cornmeal, sugar, and baking powder in a large bowl. In a medium bowl, combine milk, egg, and oil and pour into the flour mixture, stirring until moistened. Spread beef mixture in a greased 8 x 8-inch (20 x 20-cm) baking dish. Spread cornmeal mixture over the top. Bake for 10 to 12 minutes or until cornbread is done.

Nutritional Information: Calories: 669 kcal, protein: 39 g, carbohydrates: 74 g, Fat: 13 g, Cholesterol: 80 mg, Fiber: 13 g

German Meatballs

Preparation time: 10 minutes/**Cooking Time:** 40 minutes/**Total time:** 50 minutes

Servings: 6/**Difficulty Level:** Medium

Ingredients:

- 1/4 cup egg substitute
- 1/4 cup skim milk
- 1/4 cup breadcrumbs
- 1/4 teaspoon poultry seasoning
- 1-pound extra-lean ground beef (93% lean)
- 2 cups low sodium beef broth
- 1/2 cup mushrooms, sliced
- 1/2 cup onion, chopped
- 1 cup fat-free sour cream
- 1 tablespoon flour
- 1 teaspoon caraway seed

Instructions:

Combine egg substitute and milk. Stir in breadcrumbs and poultry seasoning. Add beef and mix well. Form into 24 meatballs, each about 1 1/2 inches (3.8 cm). Brown meatballs in skillet. Drain. Add broth, mushrooms, and onion to the skillet. Cover and simmer for 30 minutes. Stir together sour cream, flour, and caraway seed. Add to skillet. Cook and stir until thickened.

Nutritional Information: Calories: 281 kcal, protein: 19 g, carbohydrates: 8 g, Fat: 6 g, Cholesterol: 68 mg, Fiber: 1 g

Barbecued Beef

Preparation time: 5 minutes/**Cooking Time:** 6-8 hours on low/ 3-4 hours on high

Total time: 5-6 hours 10 minutes/**Servings:** 8/**Difficulty Level:** Medium

Ingredients:

- 1 1/2 pounds extra-lean ground beef (93% lean)
- 1 onion, chopped
- 1 cup low sodium ketchup
- 1 green bell pepper, chopped
- 2 tablespoons brown sugar
- 1/2 teaspoon garlic powder
- 2 tablespoons prepared mustard
- 3 tablespoons vinegar
- 1 tablespoon Worcestershire sauce
- 1 teaspoon chili powder

Instructions:

In a skillet, brown beef, and onion. Drain. Stir together the remaining ingredients in the slow cooker. Stir in meat and onion mixture. Cook on low for 6 to 8 hours or on high for 3 to 4 hours.

Nutritional Information: Calories: 249 kcal, protein: 17 g, carbohydrates: 12 g, Fat: 6 g, Cholesterol: 59 mg, Fiber: 0 g

Chinese Ginger Beef Stir-Fry with Baby Bok Choy

Preparation time: 10 minutes/**Cooking Time:** 15 minutes/**Total time:** 25 minutes

Servings: 4/**Difficulty Level:** Medium

Ingredients:

- 1 tablespoon of minced fresh ginger
- 12 ounces of trimmed beef flank steak,
- 1 teaspoon of dry sherry and 1 Tbsp., divided.
- 1 ½ teaspoon of soy sauce; reduced-sodium.
- 1 pound of trimmed baby bok choy, 2-inch pieces (8 cups)
- 1 teaspoon of cornstarch
- 2 tablespoons of oyster-flavored sauce,
- 1 teaspoon of toasted sesame oil
- 3 tablespoons of chicken broth; unsalted
- 1 tablespoon of vegetable oil

Instructions

Cut the beef into 2-inch-wide strips against the grain. Cut each strip into 1/4-inch-thick slices against the grain. In a medium mixing bowl, combine the 1 teaspoon sherry, ginger, beef, soy sauce, and cornstarch; whisk until the cornstarch is no more visible. Stir in the sesame oil until the meat is gently covered.

Combine the remaining 1 tablespoon of sherry in a small dish and the oyster-flavored sauce. Put it aside. Heat a 14-inch carbon-steel flat-bottomed wok (or a stainless-steel skillet of 12-inch) over the high heat until water drop vaporizes in 1 to 2 seconds. Add vegetable oil. Add the meat in a uniform layer and cook, occasionally stirring, for approximately 1 minute, or until it browns. Stir-fry for 30 seconds to 1 minute longer, until beef turns lightly browned but is not cooked through, using a metal spatula. Place on a platter to cool.

Toss in the bok choy and the broth. Cook, covered, for 1 to 2 minutes, or until the bok choy greens turns brilliant green and nearly all of the liquid has been absorbed. Return the meat to the pan, add the reserved sauce, stir-fry for 30 seconds to 1 minute, or until the bok choy is tender-crisp, and the steak is just cooked through.

Nutritional Information: Calories: 274 kcal, protein: 25.5 g, carbohydrates: 6.3 g, Fat: 1 g, Cholesterol: 68.9 mg, Fiber: 2 g

Pan-Seared Steak with Crispy Herbs & Escarole

Preparation time: 5 minutes/**Cooking Time:** 15 minutes/**Total time:** 20 minutes

Servings: 4/**Difficulty Level:** Medium

Ingredients:

- ½ teaspoon of salt, divided.
- 1 pound of sirloin steak, 1/2 inch thick
- ½ teaspoon of ground pepper, divided.
- 4 crushed cloves of garlic,
- 2 tablespoons of canola oil or grapeseed oil
- 1 sprig of fresh rosemary
- 5 sprigs of fresh thyme
- 16 cups of chopped escarole (about 1 pound)
- 3 sprigs of fresh sage

Instructions

Season the meat with a quarter teaspoon of salt and pepper. Over medium-high heat, heat a wide cast-iron skillet. Add and cook steak for 3 minutes, or until the steak is browned on one side. Add garlic, oil, sage, thyme, and rosemary to the steak and turn it over. Cook, tossing the herbs periodically, for 3 to 4 minutes, or until an instant-read thermometer placed inside the thickest part of the steak registers 125°F for medium-rare. Place the steak on a dish with the herbs and garlic on top. Make a foil tent.

Toss in the escarole and the leftover 1/4 teaspoon of salt and pepper into the pan. Cook, often stirring, for approximately 2 minutes or until the escarole begins to wilt. Serve the steak thinly sliced with crispy herbs and escarole.

Nutritional Information: Calories: 244 kcal, protein: 25.5 g, carbohydrates: 10 g, Fat: 11.8 g, Cholesterol: 59.2 mg, Fiber: 3 g

Mediterranean Brisket

Preparation time: 10 minutes/**Cooking Time:** 5 hours 30 minutes/**Total time:** 5 hrs. 40 minutes/**Servings:** 8/**Difficulty Level:** Medium

Ingredients:

- 3 teaspoons of dried crushed Italian seasoning,
- 1 3-pound of fresh beef brisket
- 2 media trimmed, fennel bulbs, cored, and cut into wedges.
- ½ cup of beef broth; lower-sodium
- 1 (14.5 ounces) can have diced no-salt-added tomatoes with garlic, basil, and oregano, undrained
- ½ cup of pitted olives
- 1 cup of Fresh Italian parsley; (flat-leaf)
- ¼ teaspoon of salt
- 1 teaspoon of lemon peel; finely shredded
- ¼ teaspoon of ground black pepper
- 2 tablespoons of all-purpose flour
- ¼ cup of cold water

Instructions

Trim any excess fat from the beef. Season it with 1 teaspoon of Italian spice. Place the meat in a slow cooker with a capacity of 3 1/2 to 4 quarts. Fennel should be sprinkled on top.

Stir broth, salt, tomatoes, olives, pepper, lemon peel, and the remaining 2 teaspoons of Italian seasoning in a mixing bowl. Pour everything into the cooker. Cook on low heat for 10-11 hours or on high heat for 5 to 5 1/2 hours, covered.

Remove the meat from the cooker and set aside the juices. Meat should be sliced. Arrange the meat and veggies on a plate and keep them warm by covering them. Skim the fat from the juices and pour them into a glass measuring cup. Then measure about 2 cups of the liquids for the sauce. Place in a saucepan. Combine the flour and cold water in a small dish; stir into the saucepan. Cook, constantly stirring until the sauce has thickened and is bubbling. Serve the sauce with the meat. Garnish with more lemon peel and parsley if desired.

Nutritional Information: Calories: 254 kcal, protein: 34.8 g, carbohydrates: 10.2 g, Fat: 8.4 g, Cholesterol: 50.6 mg, Fiber: 0.21 g

Black Skillet Beef with Greens and Red Potatoes

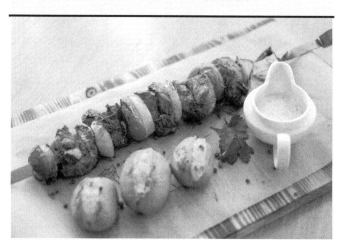

Preparation time: 10 minutes/**Cooking Time:** 40 minutes/**Total time:** 50 minutes

Servings: 6/**Difficulty Level:** Medium

Ingredients:

- 1 Tbsp. of paprika
- 1 lb. top ground beef
- 1 1/2 tsp of oregano
- 2 bunch (1/2 lb.) kale, mustard greens, or turnip greens, coarsely torn stems removed,
- 1/4 tsp of garlic powder
- 1/2 tsp of chili powder
- 1/4 tsp of black pepper
- 8 potatoes; red-skinned, halved.
- 1/8 tsp of red pepper
- 3 Cup of finely chopped onion,
- 1/8 tsp of dry mustard
- 2 Cup of beef broth
- cooking spray; nonstick as needed.
- 2 minced cloves of large garlic,
- Two large, peeled carrots, 2 1/2-inch strips

Instructions

Freeze a portion of the beef. Using a thin knife, cut long strips of 1/8-inch thick and about 3 inches wide across the grain. Paprika, chili powder, oregano, garlic powder, red pepper, black pepper, and dry mustard are combined in a bowl. Coat the meat strips with the spice mixture. Coat a big, heavy skillet with nonstick spray. Preheat the pan on high. Cook meat for 5 minutes, stirring occasionally. Then add the stock, onion, potatoes, garlic, and simmer for 20 minutes, covered, over medium heat. Stir in greens and carrots, then cover and simmer for 15 minutes, or until carrots are soft. Serve with fresh bread for dipping.

Nutritional Information: Calories: 340 kcal, protein: 30 g, carbohydrates: 45 g, Fat:5 g, Cholesterol: 64 mg, Fiber: 2.9 g

Sesame-Garlic Beef and Broccoli & Whole-Wheat Noodles

Preparation time: 35 minutes/**Cooking Time:** 30 minutes/**Total time:** 1 hour 10 minutes/**Servings:** 4/**Difficulty Level:** Medium

Ingredients:

- 2 tablespoons of soy sauce; reduced-sodium.
- 1 pound of beef sirloin steak; boneless, trimmed.
- 2 tablespoons of lemon juice
- 3 minced cloves of garlic,
- 1 tablespoon of toasted sesame oil and 2 teaspoons; divided.
- ¼ teaspoon of crushed red pepper
- 1 teaspoon of ground ginger
- 4 cups of broccoli florets
- ½ cup of water
- 6 ounces linguine; whole-wheat
- ⅛ teaspoon of ground pepper
- ½ cup of slivered onion
- Lemon wedges; for serving.
- 1 teaspoon of toasted sesame seeds

Instructions

Cut the meat into bite-size pieces by thinly slicing it against the grain. Mix the lemon juice, soy sauce, 1 tablespoon of sesame oil, garlic, ginger, and crushed red pepper in a small bowl. Pour it over the meat. Place in a shallow dish in a resealable plastic bag. Close the bag and coat it. Refrigerate the bag for 30 minutes, rotating once.

A big pot of water should be brought to a boil. Cook linguine for almost 1 minute less than the box suggests. Drain and put 1/2 cup of the cooking liquid aside.

Meanwhile, mix water and broccoli in a wok or nonstick pan and boil it over medium-high heat. Cook for 3 to 4 minutes, or until the water has evaporated. Add pepper, onion, and the remaining two tablespoons of sesame oil to a mixing bowl. Cook, stirring regularly, for 3 to 4 minutes, or until the broccoli is crisp-tender. Place the broccoli mixture in a bowl and cover with plastic wrap to keep it warm.

Drain the meat and keep the marinade aside. Add half of the meat to the heated wok (or pan) and cook, occasionally turning, for 3 to 5 minutes, or until slightly pink in the middle. Keep warm by transferring to a platter. Remove the leftover meat to a dish and repeat with the remaining beef.

In a wok (or pan), combine the leftover cooking water and marinade; add the noodles. Cook, occasionally turning, for 2 to 3 minutes over medium heat, or until noodles are cooked, and the sauce has thickened somewhat. Using 4 plates or small dishes, divide the noodle mixture. Add the meat and broccoli mixture on top. If preferred, serve with the lemon wedges and sesame seeds on top.

Nutritional Information: Calories: 357 kcal, protein: 31.1 g, carbohydrates: 39.2 g, Fat:9.7 g, Cholesterol: 59.2 mg, Fiber: 3 g

Pork Chops with Apple Cider Glaze

Preparation time: 15 minutes/**Cooking Time:** 30 minutes/**Total time:** 45 minutes

Servings: 6/**Difficulty Level:** Medium

Ingredients

- 1 tablespoon of butter
- salt and black pepper, ground; to taste.
- 1 tablespoon of vegetable oil
- ¼ cup of apple cider vinegar
- 3 minced cloves of garlic,
- 1 teaspoon of Dijon mustard
- 2 cups of apple cider
- 1 pinch of red pepper flakes
- 6 center-cut boneless pork chops (6 ounces)
- 1 teaspoon of minced rosemary

Instructions

Pork chops should be seasoned with black pepper and salt. In a big skillet, heat the oil and butter over medium-high heat. Cook each side of pork chops in the heated oil mixture for 5 to 7 minutes, or until browned on both sides and slightly pink in the middle. At least 145 degrees F should be read on an instant-read thermometer placed into the middle (63 degrees C). Remove the pork chops from the pan and place them on a platter.

Place the pan over medium-high heat and add the garlic; cook it and stir for 30 sec. Scrape off any burnt pieces from the bottom of the pan with vinegar. Add Dijon mustard and apple cider, boil it, then reduce and thicken the sauce for 3 to 4 minutes. Season them with salt and black pepper after adding the rosemary and red pepper flakes. Return the pork chops to the pan to slightly warm them up before serving, for about 1 to 2 minutes per side.

Nutritional Information: Calories: 237 kcal, protein: 21.7 g, carbohydrates: 11.8 g, Fat: 10.6 g, Cholesterol: 59.4 mg, Fiber: 3 g

Pork & Green Chile Stew

Preparation time: 10 minutes/**Cooking Time:** 4-5 hours/**Total time:** 4 hours 25 minutes/**Servings:** 6/**Difficulty Level:** Medium

Ingredients

- ½ cup of chopped onion (1 medium)
- 1 tablespoon of vegetable oil
- 3 cups of water
- 4 cups of potatoes; peeled and cubed (4 medium)
- 2 pounds of boneless pork shoulder roast or sirloin roast
- 1 (15 ounces) can of whole-kernel or hominy corn; drained
- 2 tablespoons of quick-cooking tapioca
- 2 (4 ounces) cans of undrained green chile peppers; diced
- ½ teaspoon of ancho chile powder
- ½ teaspoon of ground cumin
- One teaspoon of garlic salt
- ½ teaspoon of ground pepper
- 1 tablespoon of Chopped fresh cilantro.
- ¼ teaspoon of crushed dried oregano,

Instructions

Trim any excess fat from the meat. Using a knife, cut the pork into 1/2-inch pieces. Cook half of the meat in

heated oil over medium-high heat in a large pan. Take the meat out from the pan using a slotted spoon. Rep with the rest of the meat and onion. Remove any excess fat. Transfer the meat and onion to a slow cooker with a capacity of 3 1/2 to 4 1/2 quarts.

Add water, potatoes, hominy, ground pepper, tapioca, green chile peppers, garlic salt, ancho chile powder, cumin, and oregano. Cook covered on low for about 7 to 8 hours or on high for about 4 to 5 hours. Garnish each dish with cilantro, if preferred.

Nutritional Information: Calories: 180 kcal, protein: 15 g, carbohydrates: 22.5 g, Fat: 4.1 g, Cholesterol: 36.9 mg, Fiber: 2 g

Bavarian Beef

Preparation time: 10 minutes/**Cooking Time:** 2 hours/**Total time:** 2 hours 20 minutes/**Servings:** 5/**Difficulty Level:** Medium

Ingredients:

- 1 Tbsp of vegetable oil
- 1/8 tsp of black pepper
- 1/2 small head of red cabbage, 4 wedges
- 1 1/4 lb. of lean beef/; stew meat, remove fat: 1-inch pieces.
- 1/4 Cup of crushed gingersnaps,
- 1 large thinly sliced onion,
- 1 1/2 Cup of water
- 3/4 tsp of caraway seeds
- 1/2 tsp of salt
- 1/4 Cup of white vinegar
- 1 bay leaf
- 1 Tbsp of sugar

Instructions

In a large skillet, brown the meat in the oil. Remove the meat and cook the onion until golden in the remaining oil. Return the meat to the pan. Water, pepper, salt, caraway seeds, and bay leaf are added to the pot. Bring it to a boil. Reduce the heat to low, cover, and cook for 1 1/4 hours. Stir in the sugar and vinegar. On top of the meat, arrange the cabbage. Cover and continue to cook for another 45 minutes. Remove the meat and cabbage from the pan and place them on a plate to keep warm. Skim the fat from the drippings in the skillet. To make 1 cup of liquid, add enough water to the drippings. Add the smashed ginger snaps back to the skillet. Cook, constantly stirring until the mixture thickens and boils. Serve the sauce over the meat and veggies.

Nutritional Information: Calories: 218 kcal, protein: 24 g, carbohydrates: 14 g, Fat: 7 g, Cholesterol: 60 mg, Fiber: 1 g

Italian Pot Roast

Preparation time: 10 minutes/**Cooking Time:** 6 hours 20 minutes/**Total time:** 6 hours 35 minutes/**Servings:** 8/**Difficulty Level:** Medium

Ingredients:

- 6 whole peppercorns
- 1 cinnamon stick (3 inches)
- 3 whole allspice berries
- 4 whole cloves
- 1 (2 pounds) beef chuck roast; boneless
- 2 teaspoons of olive oil
- 2 medium sliced carrots,
- 2 sliced celery ribs,
- 4 minced garlic cloves,
- 1 large, chopped onion,
- 1 can of crushed tomatoes; (28 ounces)
- 1 cup of dry sherry or beef broth; reduced-sodium.
- Hot egg noodles; cooked and minced parsley, optional
- 1/4 teaspoon of salt

Instructions

Place the peppercorns, cloves, cinnamon stick, and allspice on a double layer of cheesecloth. To enclose the spices, gather the corners of the fabric and bind them firmly with thread.

Heat the oil in a large skillet over medium-high heat. Brown the roast on both sides and place it in a 4-quart slow cooker. Add the carrots, celery, and spice bag to the pot. In the same skillet, cook and sauté the onion until soft. Cook for a further minute after adding the garlic. Stir in the sherry to remove any browned pieces from the bottom of the pan. Bring to a boil, then reduce to 2/3 cup by cooking and stirring. Pour over the roast and veggies after adding the salt and tomatoes.

Remove the roast from the slow cooker and set it aside to keep warm. Cook for 6-7 hours on low, covered, or until veggies and meat are soft. Remove the spice bag

and skim the fat from the sauce. If preferred, serve the roast and sauce it with parsley and noodles.

Nutritional Information: Calories: 251 kcal, protein: 24 g, carbohydrates: 11 g, Fat: 12 g, Cholesterol: 74 mg, Fiber: 2 g

Beef Meatball Skewers and Cranberry Barbecue Sauce

Preparation time: 20 minutes/**Cooking Time:** 30 minutes/**Total time:** 50 minutes

Servings: 12/**Difficulty Level:** Medium

Ingredients:

- 1 pound of Ground Beef (96% lean)
- 1 cup of freshly grated zucchini
- 1/2 teaspoon of salt
- 2 trimmed red bell peppers, 1-inch pieces.
- 1 egg
- 1/4 teaspoon of pepper
- 2 trimmed green bell peppers, 1-inch pieces.
- 1 small onion, 1-inch pieces

Cranberry Barbecue Sauce

- 3 tablespoons of barbecue sauce
- 1 can (16 ounces) of cranberry sauce; whole berry

Instructions

Preheat the oven to 400 degrees Fahrenheit. Combine the salt, zucchini, egg, ground beef, and pepper in a medium mixing bowl. Mix gently but thoroughly. Shape the 24 meatballs into the size of 1-inch balls. Thread green peppers, red peppers, meatballs, and onions onto each of the twelve 6-inch skewers in random order. Place skewers on a baking sheet with a shallow rim.

Cook's Tip: To make cleanup easier, line the baking sheet with aluminum foil.

Cook for 18 to 20 minutes in a 400°F oven, or until an instant-read thermometer placed in the middle of the meatball reads 160°F.

Meanwhile, mix barbecue sauce and cranberry sauce; cook for 5 minutes or until flavors are combined. If preferred, drizzle sauce over skewers or serve as a dipping sauce.

Nutritional Information: Calories: 134 kcal, protein: 9.2 g, carbohydrates: 20 g, Fat: 2.1 g, Cholesterol: 40.5 mg, Fiber: 1 g

Chapter 15: Desserts

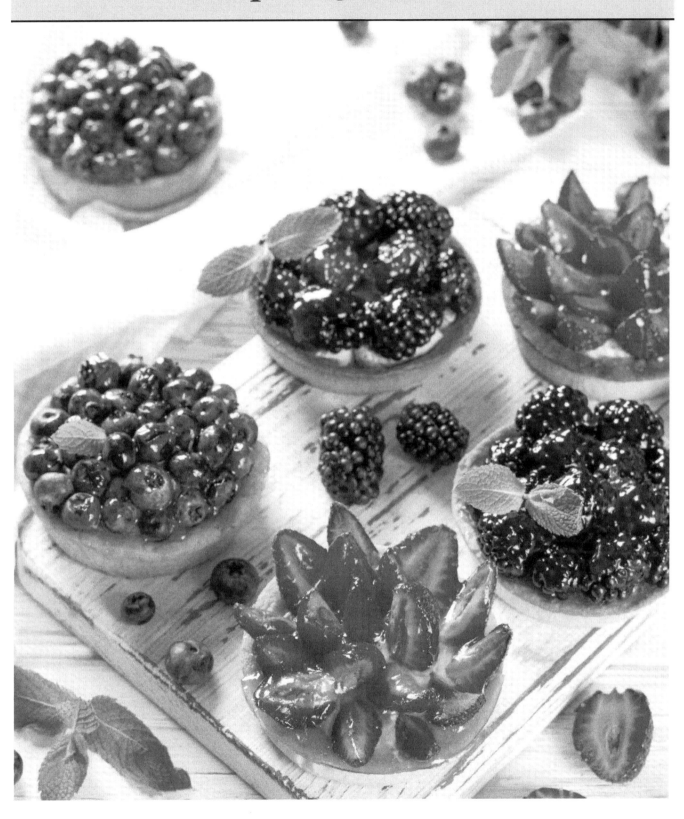

Apple Crunch

Preparation time: 10 minutes/**Cooking Time:** 35 minutes/**Total time:** 45 minutes

Servings: 6/**Difficulty Level:** Medium

Ingredients:

For Apples:

- 4 apples, peeled, cored, and chopped
- 1/2 cup sugar
- 1 teaspoon cinnamon
- 1 tablespoon unsalted margarine

For Topping:

- 1/2 cup flour
- 1/2 cup sugar
- 1 teaspoon baking powder
- 1/4 cup egg substitute
- 1/2 cup sugar
- 1 tablespoon unsalted margarine

Instructions:

Preheat an oven to 350°F (180°C, or gas mark 4) to make the apples. Mix apples, sugar, and cinnamon; pour into a greased 8 x 8-inch (20 x 20-cm) baking dish. Dot with margarine.

To make the topping: Mix topping ingredients and pour over apples. Bake for 30 to 35 minutes.

Nutritional Information: Calories: 317 kcal, protein: 3 g, carbohydrates: 70 g, Fat: 4 g, Cholesterol: 0 mg, Fiber: 2 g

Lemon pudding cakes

Preparation time: 5 minutes/**Cooking Time:** 45 minutes/**Total time:** 50 minutes

Servings: 6/**Difficulty Level:** Medium

Ingredients

- 1/4 teaspoon of salt
- 2 eggs
- 1 cup of skim milk
- 3/4 cup of sugar

- 1/3 cup of lemon juice; freshly squeezed.
- 1 tablespoon of melted butter
- 3 tablespoons of all-purpose flour
- 1 tablespoon of lemon peel; finely grated.

Instructions

Preheat the oven to 350 degrees Fahrenheit. Use cooking spray to coat 6 custard cups (6-ounce). Separate the eggs and put the whites in one mixing bowl and the yolks in another. Egg whites and salt should be whisked together at high speed in an electric mixer or stand mixer. About 1/4 cup is sugar gradually added; beat until sugar is fully dissolved and firm peaks form. Whisk egg yolks and 1/2 cup of sugar together until smooth; add milk, flour, lemon peel, lemon juice, and butter. Mix for 2 to 3 minutes, or until smooth. Gently fold the egg whites into the egg yolk mixture with a rubber spatula until just blended. Fill each custard cup halfway with the mixture. Place the custard cups in a baking pan of 13-by-9-inch and bake it. Add water to a pan and boil water until it comes halfway up to the sides of custard cups in a baking pan. Bake for about 40 to 45 minutes, or until golden and firm on top. Remove the custard cups from the oven and place them on a wire rack to cool.

Nutritional Information: Calories: 174 kcal, protein: 4 g, carbohydrates: 34 g, Fat: 4 g, Cholesterol: 68 mg, Fiber: 0.2 g

Mixed berry pie

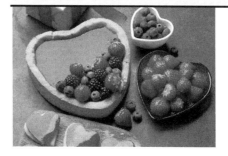

Preparation time: 5 minutes plus refrigeration time/**Cooking Time:** 0 minutes

Total time: 30 minutes/**Servings:** 6/**Difficulty Level:** Medium

Ingredients

- 3/4 cup of sliced strawberries

- 6 single-serve pie crusts; graham cracker (tart-size)
- 3/4 cup of raspberries
- 6 mint leaves; for garnish
- 1/2 cup of sugar-free, fat-free instant vanilla pudding; made of fat-free milk.
- 6 tablespoons of light whipped topping.

Instructions

Make the pudding as per package instructions. Combine the raspberries and strawberries in a small bowl.

Distribute the pudding between pie crusts (4 teaspoons). Fill each pie with approximately 2 teaspoons of the berry mixture. Add 1 tablespoon of whipped topping on top of each. Mint leaves may be used as a garnish. Serve right away or keep refrigerated.

Nutritional Information: Calories: 133 kcal, protein: 2 g, carbohydrates: 20 g, Fat: 5 g, Cholesterol: 0.5 mg, Fiber: 10.6 g

New England trifle

Preparation time: 10 minutes /**Cooking Time:** 20 minutes/**Total time:** 30 minutes

Servings: 20/**Difficulty Level:** Medium

Ingredients

- 1/4 cup of canola oil
- 1 package of yellow or white cake mix.
- 3 egg whites
- 4 cups of fresh raspberries
- 1/3 cup of frozen unsweetened concentrate orange juice; undiluted
- 6 peeled and thinly sliced peaches,
- 4 cups of fat-free milk
- 2 packages of sugar-free, fat-free instant vanilla pudding
- 1/4 cup of toasted slivered almonds,
- 1 1/4 cup of whipped light nondairy topping

Instructions

Preheat an oven to 350 degrees Fahrenheit, or the temperature indicated on the cake mix package. Use cooking spray to coat a baking pan of 17-by-11-inch lightly.

In a large mixing bowl, whisk the oil, cake mix, and egg whites with an electric blender on low speed until thoroughly combined. Fill the baking pan halfway with the cake batter. Place it in the oven and bake as directed on the box. Remove the pan from the oven and brush the warm cake with the concentrated orange juice. Allow cooling fully.

Cut the cake into 1-inch pieces and put approximately nine squares in the dish. Add cut peaches and raspberries. Whisk together the milk and vanilla pudding in a separate bowl. Pour pudding over cake and fruit. Chill the serving dishes for several hours in the refrigerator. Don't mix or stir. To serve, drizzle 1 tablespoon of whipped topping over each trifle and sprinkle almonds on top. Serve right away.

Nutritional Information: Calories: 227 kcal, protein: 4 g, carbohydrates: 37 g, Fat: traces, Cholesterol: 2 mg, Fiber: 2 g

Peach crumble

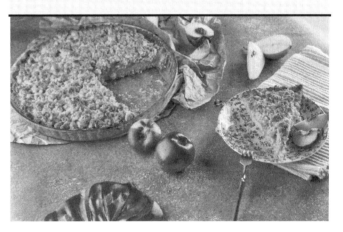

Preparation time: 10 minutes /**Cooking Time:** 20 minutes/**Total time:** 30 minutes

Servings: 8/**Difficulty Level:** Medium

Ingredients

- Juice from one lemon
- 8 ripe peeled, pitted sliced freestone peaches,
- 1/4 teaspoon of ground nutmeg
- 1/3 teaspoon of ground cinnamon
- 1/4 cup of dark brown sugar; packed.
- 1/2 cup of whole-wheat flour
- 1/4 cup of quick-cooking oats

- 2 tablespoons of margarine; trans-free, thin slices

Instructions

Preheat an oven to 375 degrees Fahrenheit. Coat a 9-inch pie tin lightly with cooking spray.

Place peach slices in a pie dish that has been prepared. Lemon juice, nutmeg, and cinnamon are sprinkled over the top. Put them aside.

Combine brown sugar and flour in a small mixing dish. Cut margarine and mix it into the flour-sugar mixture using your fingertips. Stir in the uncooked oats until they are equally distributed. On top of the peaches, sprinkle the flour mixture. Bake for 30 minutes, or until the peaches are tender and the topping turns golden. Serve warm, cut into 8 pieces

Nutritional Information: Calories: 137 kcal, protein: 3 g, carbohydrates: 26 g, Fat: 4 g, Cholesterol: 0 mg, Fiber: 3.4 g

Sauteed bananas

Preparation time: 30 minutes /**Cooking Time:** 30 minutes/**Total time:** 60 minutes

Servings: 6/**Difficulty Level:** Medium

Ingredients

For the sauce:

- 1 tablespoon of honey
- 1 tablespoon of walnut oil
- 2 tablespoons of brown sugar; firmly packed
- 1 tablespoon of golden raisins or dark raisins (sultanas)
- 1 tablespoon of butter
- 3 tablespoons of 1 percent milk; low-fat

For the sauté:

- 2 tablespoons of dark rum
- 1/2 teaspoon of canola oil
- 4 firm bananas; about 1 pound

Instructions

Begin by preparing the sauce. Melt the butter in a small saucepan over medium heat. Add honey, walnut oil, and brown sugar. Cook, constantly stirring, for 3 minutes, or until the sugar has dissolved. Cook, constantly stirring, until the sauce thickens slightly, for approximately 3 minutes after adding 1 tablespoon of milk at a time. Remove the pan from heat and add the raisins. Remove from the oven and keep warm.

Peel the bananas and cut each one into three pieces crosswise. Each piece should be cut in half lengthwise. Place a nonstick large frying pan over medium-high heat and lightly cover with canola oil. Add bananas and cook for 3 to 4 minutes or brown. Keep warm by transferring to a platter.

Add rum to the pan, get it to a boil, and deglaze the pan, scraping up any browned pieces from the bottom with a wooden spoon. Cook for 30 to 45 seconds, or until the liquid has been reduced by half. To reheat the bananas, return them to the pan.

Divide the bananas into separate dishes or plates to serve. Serve immediately with the heated sauce drizzled over the top.

Nutritional Information: Calories: 145 kcal, protein: 1 g, carbohydrates: 27 g, Fat: 5 g, Cholesterol: 5 mg, Fiber: 2.4 g

Banana Mousse

Preparation time: 5 minutes /**Cooking Time:** 0 minutes/**Total time:** 10 minutes

Servings: 4/**Difficulty Level:** Easy

Ingredients

- 1 tsp of vanilla
- 4 tsp of sugar
- 1 medium banana; quarters
- 8 slices of banana (1/4 inch)
- 2 Tbsp of low-fat milk
- 1 Cup of low-fat plain yogurt

Instructions

Combine the vanilla, sugar, milk, and banana in a blender. Process at high speed for 15 seconds or until smooth. Pour the mixture into a small mixing dish and stir in the yogurt. Chill. Before serving, spoon into 4 dessert plates and top with two banana slices for each.

Nutritional Information: Calories: 94 kcal, protein: 1 g, carbohydrates: 18 g, Fat: 1 g, Cholesterol: 4 mg, Fiber: 1.4 g

Wacky chocolate cake

Preparation time: 5 minutes /**Cooking Time:** 35 minutes/**Total time:** 40 minutes

Servings: 18/**Difficulty Level:** Medium

Ingredients

- 3 tbsps. of cocoa powder; unsweetened
- 1 cup of sugar
- 2 1/4 teaspoons of baking soda
- 3 cups of pastry flour; whole-wheat
- 1/2 teaspoon of salt
- 2 tablespoons of vinegar
- 1 tablespoon of vanilla
- 2 cups of water
- 1/2 cup of canola oil

Instructions

Preheat an oven to 350 degrees Fahrenheit. In a 9-by-13-inch ungreased baking pan, combine sugar, flour, salt, cocoa powder, and baking soda. Toss them together with a whisk.

Make three holes in the dry mixture using a spoon. Pour the vanilla extract into one of the holes. Fill another hole with vinegar. Fill the third hole with oil.

Microwave the water for 3 minutes on high, or until it boils. Pour boiling water over the contents in the pan gently and evenly. Mix them for about 2 minutes with the whisk. There should be no traces of dry ingredients left.

Bake for 25–30 minutes, or until the tester inserted in the middle comes out clean. Allow the cake to finish cooking. Serve after cutting into 18 squares.

Nutritional Information: Calories: 183 kcal, protein: 3 g, carbohydrates: 27 g, Fat: 7 g, Cholesterol: 0 mg, Fiber: 1 g

Vanilla poached peaches

Preparation time: 5 minutes /**Cooking Time:** 15 minutes/**Total time:** 20 minutes

Servings: 4/**Difficulty Level:** Medium

Ingredients

- 1/2 cup of sugar
- 1 cup of water
- 1 split and scraped vanilla bean,
- Mint leaves /cinnamon; for garnish
- 4 large pitted and quartered peaches,

Instructions

Combine the vanilla bean, sugar, water, and scrapings in a saucepan. Stir the mixture over low heat until the sugar melts. Continue to cook, occasionally stirring, until the mixture thickens; it will take approximately 10 minutes.

Fill tiny ornamental dishes halfway with peaches and sauce. Toss in the chopped fruit. Cook for approximately 5 minutes over low heat. Mint leaves and a sprinkling of cinnamon may be used as a garnish. Serve right away.

Nutritional Information: Calories: 156 kcal, protein: 1 g, carbohydrates: 38 g, Fat: traces, Cholesterol: 0 mg, Fiber: 2 g

Berry Cobbler

Preparation time: 10 minutes /**Cooking Time:** 35 minutes/**Total time:** 45 minutes

Servings: 8/**Difficulty Level:** Medium

Ingredients

- 2 tablespoons cornstarch
- 1/2 cup water, divided
- 1 1/2 cups sugar, divided
- 1 tablespoon lemon juice
- 1 teaspoon baking powder
- 4 cups blackberries
- 1 cup flour
- 3 tablespoons unsalted margarine

Instructions

Preheat oven to 400°F (200°C, or gas mark 6). In a saucepan, stir together the cornstarch and 1/4 cup (60 ml) cold water until cornstarch is completely dissolved. Add 1 cup (200 g) sugar, lemon juice, and blackberries; combine gently. Combine the flour, remaining sugar, and baking powder in a bowl. Blend in the margarine until the mixture resembles a coarse meal. Boil the remaining 1/4 cup (60 ml) water and stir into the flour mixture until it just forms a dough. Transfer the blackberry mixture to a 1 1/2-quart (1.4-L) baking dish. Drop spoonsful of the dough carefully onto the berries and bake the cobbler on a baking sheet in the middle of the oven for 20 to 25 minutes, or until the topping is golden.

Nutritional Information: Calories: 280 kcal, protein: 3 g, carbohydrates: 59 g, Fat: 5 g, Cholesterol: 0 mg, Fiber: 4 g

Apple Tapioca

Preparation time: 5 minutes /**Cooking Time:** 3-4 hours/**Total time:** 4 hours 5 minutes/**Servings:** 4/**Difficulty Level:** Medium

Ingredients

- 4 cups apples, peeled and sliced
- 1/2 cup brown sugar
- 3/4 teaspoon cinnamon
- 2 tablespoons tapioca
- 2 tablespoons lemon juice
- 1 cup boiling water

Instructions

Toss apples with brown sugar, cinnamon, and tapioca in a medium bowl until evenly coated. Place apples in a slow cooker. Pour lemon juice over the top. Pour in boiling water. Cook on high for 3 to 4 hours.

Nutritional Information: Calories: 176 kcal, protein: 0 g, carbohydrates: 46 g, Fat: 0 g, Cholesterol: 0 mg, Fiber: 2 g

Sweet Potato Pudding

Preparation time: 10 minutes /**Cooking Time:** 50 minutes/**Total time:** 60 minutes

Servings: 8/**Difficulty Level:** Medium

Ingredients

- 4 cups cooked and mashed sweet potatoes
- 3/4 cup sugar
- 1/2 cup egg substitute
- 1/2 cup coconut milk
- 1 tablespoon lime juice
- 1/4 cup rum
- 1/2 teaspoon baking powder
- 1/2 teaspoon cinnamon
- 1/4 cup raisins

Instructions

Preheat an oven to 350°F (180°C, or gas mark 4). To mashed potatoes, alternate adding sugar and egg substitute, mixing well after each addition. Add coconut milk. Blend well. Mix in lime juice and rum. Mix well. Combine baking powder and cinnamon and add to potato mixture, along with raisins. Mix well. Pour mixture into a greased tube cake or Bundt pan and bake for 50 minutes, or until done.

Nutritional Information: Calories: 271 kcal, protein: 5 g, carbohydrates: 53 g, Fat: 4 g, Cholesterol: 0 mg, Fiber: 4 g

Honey Grilled Apples

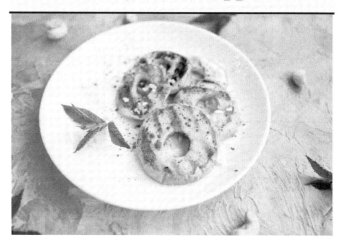

Preparation time: 10 minutes /**Cooking Time:** 20 minutes/**Total time:** 30 minutes

Servings: 4/**Difficulty Level:** Easy

Ingredients

- 4 apples
- 1 tablespoon honey
- 2 tablespoons lemon juice
- 1 tablespoon unsalted margarine

Instructions

Core apples and cut slices through the skin to make each apple resemble orange sections. Mix the honey, lemon juice, and margarine. Spoon mixture into apple cores. Wrap apples in greased heavy-duty aluminum foil, fold up and seal. Grill until tender, about 20 minutes.

Nutritional Information: Calories: 104 kcal, protein: 0 g, carbohydrates: 21 g, Fat: 3 g, Cholesterol: 0 mg, Fiber: 2 g

Pumpkin Cookies

Preparation time: 10 minutes /**Cooking Time:** 15 minutes/**Total time:** 30 minutes

Servings: 30/**Difficulty Level:** Easy

Ingredients

- 1 teaspoon of baking powder
- 2 cups of flour
- 1/2 teaspoon of baking soda
- 1 teaspoon cinnamon
- 1/4 cup canola oil
- 1/2 teaspoon of ground ginger
- 6 tablespoons egg substitute
- 1 teaspoon of ground allspice
- 1 cup packed brown sugar
- 1 cup canned or cooked fresh pumpkin
- 1 teaspoon vanilla

Instructions

Preheat an oven to 350°F (180°C, or gas mark 4). Combine flour, baking soda, ginger, cinnamon, baking powder, and allspice in a medium bowl. Beat oil, brown sugar, egg substitute, pumpkin, and vanilla in a wide bowl. Stir flour mixture into wet ingredients until just combined. Drop spoonsful of dough about 1 inch (2.5 cm) apart on an ungreased baking sheet. Bake for 12 to 14 minutes.

Nutritional Information: Calories: 81 kcal, protein: 1 g, carbohydrates: 14 g, Fat: 2 g, Cholesterol: 0 mg, Fiber: 1 g

Cookies and cream shake

Preparation time: 15 minutes /**Cooking Time:** 0 minutes/**Total time:** 15 minutes

Servings: 3/**Difficulty Level:** Easy

Ingredients

- 6 crushed chocolate wafer cookies,
- 3 cups of vanilla ice cream; fat-free
- 1 1/3 cups of chilled vanilla soy milk; (soya milk),

Instructions

Combine ice cream and soy milk in a blender. Blend until the mixture is smooth and foamy. Toss in the cookies and pulse a few times to combine. Immediately pour into tall, cold glasses and serve.

Nutritional Information: Calories: 270 kcal, protein: 9 g, carbohydrates: 52 g, Fat: 3 g, Cholesterol: traces, Fiber: 1 g

Dessert Pizza

Preparation time: 10 minutes /**Cooking Time:** 30 minutes/**Total time:** 40 minutes

Servings: 16/**Difficulty Level:** Medium

Ingredients

- 1/2 cup unsalted margarine
- 3/4 cup brown sugar
- 1 egg yolk
- 1 teaspoon vanilla
- 1 1/2 cups flour
- 1 1/4 cups chocolate chips
- 1 1/2 cups miniature marshmallows
- 1/2 cup dry-roasted peanuts, chopped

Instructions

Preheat oven to 350°F (180°C, or gas mark 4). Beat the margarine in a large mixing bowl with an electric mixer on medium-high speed for 30 seconds. Add brown sugar and beat until combined. Beat in egg yolk and vanilla until combined. Beat in as much of the flour as you can with the mixer. Stir in any remaining flour with a wooden spoon. Spread dough in a lightly greased 12-inch (30-cm) pizza pan. Bake for 25 minutes, or until golden. Sprinkle hot crust with the chocolate chips. Let stand for 1 to 2 minutes to soften. Spread chocolate over crust. Sprinkle with marshmallows and nuts. Bake for 3 minutes more or until marshmallows are puffed and brown. Cool in pan on a wire rack.

Nutritional Information: Calories: 247 kcal, protein: 4 g, carbohydrates: 32 g, Fat: 12 g, Cholesterol: 16 mg, Fiber: 1 g

Lemon Biscotti

Preparation time: 10 minutes /**Cooking Time:** 40 minutes/**Total time:** 50 minutes

Servings: 24/**Difficulty Level:** Medium

Ingredients

- 1 1/2 teaspoons lemon juice
- 2 1/2 cups flour
- 1 teaspoon of baking powder
- 3/4 cup sugar
- 1 teaspoon baking soda
- 1 cup egg substitute
- 1 tablespoon lemon zest

Instructions

Preheat oven to 325°F (170°C, or gas mark 3). Sift together flour, baking powder, and baking soda. In another bowl, beat egg substitute and sugar together; TIP: If you're not into dunking and want a softer cookie, reduce the second baking time to 10 minutes. Then beat in lemon zest and lemon juice. Add flour mixture to egg mixture and stir until well mixed. On a floured surface, knead the dough for 2 minutes. Divide dough in half and shape into 2 logs, about 1 inch (2.5 cm) high and 4 inches (10 cm) wide. Bake for 30 minutes, or until golden brown. Remove from oven and cool. Reduce oven temperature to 300°F (150°C, or gas mark 2). Slice logs diagonally into 1/2-inch (1.3-cm) thick slices and put slices back on a baking sheet, cut side down. Bake for another 20 minutes.

Nutritional Information: Calories: 81 kcal, protein: 3 g, carbohydrates: 16 g, Fat: 0 g, Cholesterol: 0 mg, Fiber: 0 g

Orange slices and citrus syrup

Preparation time: 25 minutes plus chill time /**Cooking Time:** 15 minutes

Total time: 4 hours/**Servings:** 4/**Difficulty Level:** Medium

Ingredients

- Zest of one orange, thin strips 1/8-inch-wide and 4 inches long
- 4 oranges

For syrup:

- 2 tablespoons of dark honey
- 1 1/2 cups of fresh strained orange juice,

For garnish:

- 4 mint sprigs; fresh
- 2 tablespoons of orange liqueur; Cointreau or Grand Marnier (optional)

Instructions

Cut a small slice from the top and bottom of each orange, exposing the flesh, one at a time. Placing the orange upright, take off the peel by following the shape of the fruit, remove all of the white pith and membrane with a sharp knife. Cut the orange into 1/2-inch-thick slices crosswise. Transfer to a nonaluminum shallow bowl or dish. Carry on with the other remaining oranges in the same manner and set them aside.

Combine the strips of zest with enough water to cover in a small saucepan over medium-high heat. Bring to a boil, then reduce to a simmer for 1 minute. Drain the zest and place it in a bowl of cold water. Set it aside. Mix the honey and orange juice in a wide saucepan over medium-high heat to create the syrup. Boil it, constantly stirring to ensure that the honey is completely dissolved. Reduce the heat to medium-low and cook, uncovered, for approximately 5 minutes, or until the mixture forms a light syrup. Add the orange zest to the syrup after draining it. Cook for 3 to 5 minutes, or until zest is translucent. Over the oranges, pour the mixture. Cover and chill for up to three hours, or until well cooled. Divide the orange segments and syrup amongst separate dishes to serve. If using, drizzle 1 1/2 tsp of orange liqueur over each serving. Serve immediately with a mint garnish.

Nutritional Information: Calories: 182 kcal, protein: 2 g, carbohydrates: 39 g, Fat: < 1g, Cholesterol: 0 mg, Fiber: 4 g

Fruitcake

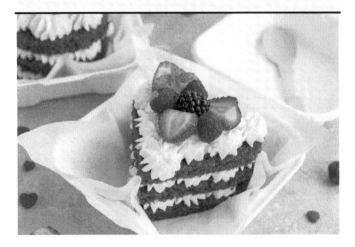

Preparation time: 10 minutes /**Cooking Time:** 60 minutes/**Total time:** 1 hour 10 minutes/**Servings:** 12/**Difficulty Level:** Medium

Ingredients

- 1/2 cup of unsweetened applesauce
- 2 cups of assorted dried chopped fruit, such as dates, currants, cherries, or figs
- 1/2 cup of pineapple stored in juice; crushed, drained.
- 2 tablespoons of real vanilla extract
- Zest and juice of one medium orange
- 1/2 cup of unsweetened apple juice
- 1/2 cup of chopped or crushed walnuts zest and juice of one lemon
- 1/2 cup of rolled oats.
- 1/4 cup of sugar
- 1 cup of pastry flour; whole-wheat
- 1/4 cup of flaxseed flour
- 1/2 teaspoon of baking powder
- 1 egg
- 1/2 teaspoon of baking soda

Instructions

Combine the applesauce, dried fruit, fruit zests, pineapple, juices, and vanilla in a medium mixing bowl. Allow 15 to 20 mins to soak. Using parchment (baking) paper, line the base of a 9-inch-by-4-inch pan.

Whisk baking soda, oats, sugar, flour, and baking powder in a large mixing bowl. Stir together the fruit and liquid combined with the dry ingredients. Add walnuts and egg to a mixing bowl.

Fill the loaf pan halfway with batter and bake for one hour, or until the toothpick inserted in the middle comes out clean. Allow the fruitcake to cool in the pan for 30 mins before removing it.

Nutritional Information: Calories: 229 kcal, protein: 5 g, carbohydrates: 41 g, Fat: 5 g, Cholesterol: 41 mg, Fiber: 1 g

Fruited rice pudding

Preparation time: 10 minutes /**Cooking Time:** 50 minutes/**Total time:** 60 minutes

Servings: 8/**Difficulty Level:** Easy

Ingredients

- 1 cup of brown rice; long-grain
- 2 cups of water
- 1/2 cup of brown sugar
- 4 cups of fat-free milk
- 1 teaspoon of vanilla extract
- 1/2 teaspoon of lemon zest
- 1/4 cup of crushed pineapple
- 6 egg whites
- 1/4 cup of chopped dried apricots,
- 1/4 cup of raisins

Instructions

Boil 2 cups of water in a saucepan. Cook for 10 minutes after adding the rice. Fill a colander halfway with water and drain completely.

Add brown sugar and evaporated milk in the same pot. Cook until heated. Add lemon zest, cooked rice, and vanilla essence. Simmer for 30 minutes over low heat or until the stew is thick and rice is soft. Remove from the heat and set aside to cool.

Whisk the egg whites together in a small dish. Pour it over the rice mixture. Add raisins, pineapple, and apricots. Stir until everything is thoroughly combined.

Preheat the oven to 325 degrees Fahrenheit. Fill the baking dish halfway with the pudding and fruit mixture. Using cooking spray, lightly coat the baking dish. Bake for 20 minutes or until the pudding is set. Warm or chilly is OK.

Nutritional Information: Calories: 257 kcal,

protein: 17 g, carbohydrates: 48 g, Fat: 1 g, Cholesterol: 5 mg, Fiber: 2.7 g

Lemon cheesecake

Preparation time: 10 minutes /**Cooking Time:** 20 minutes/**Total time:** 30 minutes

Servings: 8/**Difficulty Level:** Easy

Ingredients

- 1 envelope of unflavored gelatin
- 2 tablespoons of cold water
- 1/2 cup of skim milk; heat to boiling point
- 2 tablespoons of lemon juice
- Egg substitute equal to one egg or two egg whites
- 1 teaspoon of vanilla
- 1/4 cup of sugar
- Lemon zest
- 2 cups of low-fat cottage cheese

Instructions

Combine the gelatin, water, and lemon juice in a blender container. The process is for 1 to 2 minutes at low speed to soften gelatin.

Add the boiling milk and process until the gelatin is completely dissolved. Add egg replacement, vanilla, sugar, and cheese in a blender container, and blend until smooth.

Fill a 9-inch pie pan or a circular flat dish halfway with the mixture. Refrigerate for 2 to 3 hours. Just before serving, sprinkle with lemon zest if desired.

Nutritional Information: Calories: 80 kcal, protein: 9 g, carbohydrates: 9 g, Fat: 1 g, Cholesterol: 3 mg, Fiber: 0.2 g

Whole-grain mixed berry coffeecake

Preparation time: 10 minutes /**Cooking Time:** 30 minutes/**Total time:** 40 minutes

Servings: 8/**Difficulty Level:** Easy

Ingredients

- 1 tablespoon of vinegar
- 1/2 cup of skim milk
- 1 teaspoon of vanilla
- 2 tablespoons of canola oil
- 1/3 cup of packed brown sugar
- 1 egg
- 1/2 teaspoon of ground cinnamon
- 1 cup of pastry flour; whole-wheat
- 1/2 teaspoon of baking soda
- 1/8 teaspoon of salt
- 1/4 cup of low-fat slightly crushed granola,
- 1 cup of frozen mixed berries, such as raspberries, blueberries, and blackberries

Instructions

Preheat the oven to 350 degrees Fahrenheit. Use a cooking spray to coat a cake pan or 8-inch round and coat it with flour.

Combine the vinegar, milk, oil, egg, vanilla, and brown sugar in a large mixing bowl and whisk until smooth. Just until moistened, stir in flour, cinnamon, baking soda, and salt. Fold half of the berries into the batter gently. Pour into the pan that has been prepared. Lastly, top with the granola and remaining berries.

Bake for 25 to 30 minutes, or until golden brown and the center of the top snaps back when touched. Cool for 10 minutes in the pan on a cooling rack. Warm the dish before serving.

Nutritional Information: Calories: 165 kcal, protein: 4 g, carbohydrates: 26 g, Fat: 5 g, Cholesterol: 24 mg, Fiber: 3 g

Almond & apricot biscotti

Preparation time: 20 minutes /**Cooking Time:** 60 minutes/**Total time:** 1 hour 20 minutes/**Servings:** 24/**Difficulty Level:** Medium

Ingredients:

- 1/4 cup of brown sugar; firmly packed
- 2 lightly beaten eggs,
- 1 teaspoon of baking powder
- 3/4 cup of all-purpose flour (plain)
- 2 tablespoons of low-fat 1 percent milk
- 1/2 teaspoon of almond extract
- 2 tablespoons of canola oil
- 1/4 cup of coarsely chopped almonds.
- 2 tablespoons of dark honey
- 3/4 cup of whole-wheat flour; (whole-meal)

- 2/3 cup of dried apricots; chopped.

Instructions

Preheat an oven to 350 degrees Fahrenheit. Combine the brown sugar, flours, and baking powder in a large mixing bowl. To combine ingredients, whisk them together. Add the milk, eggs, honey, canola oil, and almond extract to a mixing bowl. Stir the dough with the wooden spoon until it barely comes together. Add chopped apricots and almonds. Mix until the dough is well-blended using floured hands.

Shape the dough into a flattened log 3 inches wide, 12 inches long, and approximately 1-inch-high on a long piece of plastic and wrap by hand. Transfer the dough to a nonstick baking sheet by lifting the plastic wrap. Bake for 25 to 30 minutes, or until gently browned. Allow it cool for 10 minutes on another baking sheet.

On a cutting board, place the cooled log. Cut 24 1/2-inch broad slices diagonally crosswise using a serrated knife. Arrange the slices on the baking sheet, cut-side down. Put it back in the oven and bake for 15 to 20 minutes, or until crisp. Allow cooling fully before transferring to a wire rack. Keep the container sealed.

Nutritional Information: Calories: 75 kcal, protein: 2 g, carbohydrates: 12 g, Fat: 2 g, Cholesterol: 15 mg, Fiber: 1 g

Apple dumplings

Preparation time: 2 hours /**Cooking Time:** 30 minutes/**Total time:** 2 hours 30 minutes/**Servings:** 8/**Difficulty Level:** Medium

Ingredients:

Dough:

- 2 tablespoons of apple liquor or brandy
- 1 tablespoon of butter
- 2 tablespoons of buckwheat flour
- 1 teaspoon of honey
- 2 tablespoons of rolled oats.
- 1 cup of whole-wheat flour

Apple filling:

- 1 teaspoon of nutmeg
- 6 large thinly sliced tart apples,
- Zest of 1 lemon

- 2 tablespoons of honey

Instructions

Preheat an oven to 350 degrees Fahrenheit. Combine the flours, honey, butter, and oats in a food processor. Pulse a few times more until the mixture resembles a fine meal. Pulse a few more times to incorporate the brandy or apple liquor until the mixture begins to form a ball. Refrigerate it for two hours after removing the mixture from the food processor. Combine nutmeg, apples, and honey. Toss in the lemon zest. Set it aside.

Extra flour is used to roll out the chilled dough to a thickness of 1/4 inch. Using an 8-inch circle cutter, cut the dough into 8-inch circles. Use an 8-cup muffin pan that has been gently sprayed with cooking spray. Place a dough circle over each gently sprayed cup. Gently press dough into place. Fill them with the apple mixture. To seal, fold over the edges, squeeze the top, and bake for 30 minutes or golden brown.

Nutritional Information: Calories: 178 kcal, protein: 3 g, carbohydrates: 36 g, Fat: 2.5 g, Cholesterol: 4 mg, Fiber: 1 g

Carrot & spice quick bread

Preparation time: 15 minutes/**Cooking Time:** 45 minutes/**Total time:** 60 minutes

Servings: 17/**Difficulty Level:** Medium

Ingredients:

- cup of whole-wheat flour

- teaspoon of grated orange rind

- 1/2 cup of all-purpose flour; sifted.

- tablespoon of walnuts; finely chopped.

- 1/4 cup and 2 tablespoons of brown sugar; firmly packed

- 1/2 teaspoon of ground cinnamon

- 1 1/2 cups of shredded carrots

- 1/4 teaspoon of ground ginger

- tablespoons of golden raisins

- 1/2 teaspoon of baking soda

- 1/3 cup of skim milk

- beaten egg whites/ egg substitute equal to 1 egg,

- 1 teaspoon of vanilla extract

- tablespoons of unsweetened orange juice

- 1/3 cup of margarine; trans-fat-free, softened.

- teaspoons of baking powder

Instructions

Preheat the oven to 375 degrees Fahrenheit. Cooking spray coats a 2 ½ by 4 ½ by 8 ½ inch loaf pan.

Combine the dry ingredients: flours, baking soda, powder, cinnamon, and ginger in a small dish and set them aside.

In a large mixing bowl, blend margarine and sugar using an electric mixer or by hand. Add orange juice, milk, vanilla, egg, and orange rind in a mixing bowl. Stir in raisins, carrots, and walnuts in a mixing bowl. Add dry ingredients that have been set aside. Mix thoroughly.

Preheat the oven to 350°F and bake for about 45 mins, or until a wooden pick inserted in the middle comes out clean. Pour the batter into the loaf pan. Allow 10 minutes to cool in the pan. Remove the pan from the oven and cool fully on a wire rack.

Nutritional Information: Calories: 110 kcal, protein: 2 g, carbohydrates: 15 g, Fat: 5 g, Cholesterol: traces, Fiber: 1 g

Grapes and lemon sour cream sauce

Preparation time: 10 minutes/**Cooking Time:** 0 minutes/**Total time:** 20 minutes

Servings: 6/**Difficulty Level:** Medium

Ingredients:

- 2 tablespoons of powdered sugar
- 1/2 cup of sour cream; fat-free
- 1/2 teaspoon of lemon zest
- 1/8 teaspoon of vanilla extract
- 1/2 teaspoon of lemon juice
- 1 1/2 cups of seedless red grapes
- 3 tablespoons of chopped walnuts
- 1 1/2 cups of seedless green grapes

Instructions

Combine lemon juice, powdered sugar, sour cream, lemon zest, and vanilla in a small mixing bowl. To ensure an equal distribution of ingredients, whisk them together. Refrigerate for several hours after covering.

In six stemmed dessert cups or bowls, place equal parts of grapes, top each dish with a dollop of sauce and 1/2 spoonful of chopped walnuts. Serve right away.

Nutritional Information: Calories: 106 kcal, protein: 2 g, carbohydrates: 208 g, Fat: 2 g, Cholesterol: 2 mg, Fiber: 1 g

Orange dream smoothie

Preparation time: 10 minutes/**Cooking Time:** 0 minutes/**Total time:** 10 minutes

Servings: 4/**Difficulty Level:** Medium

Ingredients:

- 1 1/2 cups of chilled orange juice,
- 1 teaspoon of grated orange zest
- 1 cup of soy milk; light vanilla, chilled
- 1/3 cup of soft or silken tofu
- 1 tablespoon of dark honey
- 1/2 teaspoon of vanilla extract
- 4 peeled orange segments
- 5 ice cubes

Instructions

Blend the blender with soy milk, orange juice, vanilla, tofu, orange zest, honey, and ice cubes. Blend for approximately 30 seconds or until smooth and foamy.

Pour into long chilled glasses, and with an orange

segment, garnish each glass.

Nutritional Information: Calories: 101 kcal, protein: 3 g, carbohydrates: 20 g, Fat: 1 g, Cholesterol: 0 mg, Fiber: 1 g

Rustic apple-cranberry tart

Preparation time: 10 minutes/**Cooking Time:** 50 minutes/**Total time:** 2 hours

Servings: 8/**Difficulty Level:** Medium

Ingredients:

For the filling:

- 1/4 cup of apple juice
- 1/2 cup of dried cranberries
- 1/4 teaspoon of ground cinnamon
- 2 tablespoons of cornstarch
- 1 teaspoon of vanilla extract
- 4 large cored, peeled, sliced tart apples,

For the crust:

- 2 teaspoons of sugar
- 1 1/4 cups of whole-wheat flour(whole-meal)
- 1/4 cup of ice water
- 3 tablespoons of trans-free margarine

Instructions

Combine the apple juice and cranberries in a small microwave-safe bowl. Cook for 1 minute on high, then stir. Cover and leave aside for 1 hour, or until mixture is near to room temperature. Continue to cook the apple juice for 30 sec at a time, tossing after each interval, until it is extremely warm.

Preheat an oven to 375 degrees Fahrenheit. Combine the apple slices and cornstarch in a large mixing bowl. Toss well to get an equal coating. Add juice and cranberries to a mixing bowl. Mix thoroughly. Add cinnamon and vanilla to a mixing bowl. Put it aside.

In a large mixing bowl, combine flour and sugar to make the crust. Add sliced margarine into the mixture and mix well until crumbly. Add one tablespoon of ice water and stir with a fork until the dough forms a rough lump.

Place a big sheet of aluminum foil on the surface and tape it down. It should be dusted with flour. Flatten the dough in the middle of the foil. Roll the dough from the center to the edges with a rolling pin to form a 13-inch-diameter circle. Add fruit filling in the dough's middle. Cover the dough with the filling, leaving about a 1- to 2-inch border. Fold the crust's top and bottom edges up over the filling. The pastry will not completely cover the contents; it should have a rustic appearance.

Remove the foil and the countertop from the tape. Cover the tart with another piece of foil to cover the exposed fruit. Slide the tart onto a baking sheet, top and bottom foil included, and bake for 30 minutes. Remove the foil from the top and bake for another 10 minutes or browned. Serve immediately after cutting into 8 wedges.

Nutritional Information: Calories: 197 kcal, protein: 3 g, carbohydrates: 35 g, Fat: 5 g, Cholesterol: 0 mg, Fiber: 5 g

Strawberries and cream

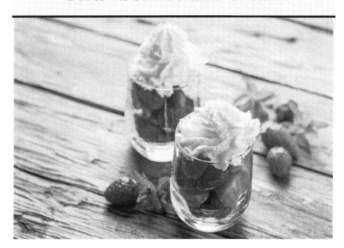

Preparation time: 10 minutes/**Cooking Time:** 0 minutes/**Total time:** 1 hour 10 minutes /**Servings:** 6/**Difficulty Level:** Medium

Ingredients:

- 1/2 cup of brown sugar
- 1 1/2 cups of sour cream; fat-free
- 1 quart fresh hulled and halved strawberries; (6 whole for garnish)
- 2 tablespoons of amaretto liqueur

Instructions

Whisk the brown sugar, sour cream, and liqueur in a small bowl.

Combine the sour cream mixture and halved strawberries in a large mixing bowl. To combine, carefully stir everything together. Cover and chill for 1 hour or until well cooked.

Fill 6 chilled sherbet glasses or colored bowls halfway with strawberries. Serve immediately with whole strawberries as a garnish.

Nutritional Information: Calories: 136 kcal, protein: 3 g, carbohydrates: 31 g, Fat: traces, Cholesterol: 6 mg, Fiber: 5 g

Whole-grain banana bread

Preparation time: 20 minutes/**Cooking Time:** 60 minutes/**Total time:** 1 hour 20 minutes /**Servings:** 14 /**Difficulty Level:** Medium

Ingredients:

- 1/2 cup of amaranth flour
- 1/2 cup of brown rice flour
- 1/2 cup of millet flour
- 1/2 cup of tapioca flour
- 1 teaspoon of baking soda
- 1/2 cup of quinoa flour
- 1/8 teaspoon of salt
- 1/2 teaspoon of baking powder
- 2 tablespoons of grapeseed oil
- 3/4 cup of egg substitute/ (egg whites)
- 2 cups of mashed banana
- 1/2 cup of raw sugar

Instructions

Preheat an oven to 350 degrees Fahrenheit. Spray a 5-by-9-inch loaf pan lightly with cooking spray before using. Sprinkle with a pinch of flour. Put it aside.

Combine all dry ingredients (excluding sugar) in a large mixing bowl. Combine oil, sugar, egg, and mashed banana in a separate bowl. Mix thoroughly. Combine the wet and dry ingredients in a large mixing bowl. Fill the loaf pan halfway with batter and bake for 50–60 minutes.

Check the doneness with a toothpick – there should be no batter stuck to it when you remove it. Remove the bread from the oven when done, let it cool, then slice and serve.

Nutritional Information: Calories: 163 kcal, protein: 4 g, carbohydrates: 30 g, Fat: 3 g, Cholesterol: 0 mg g, Fiber: 4.5 g

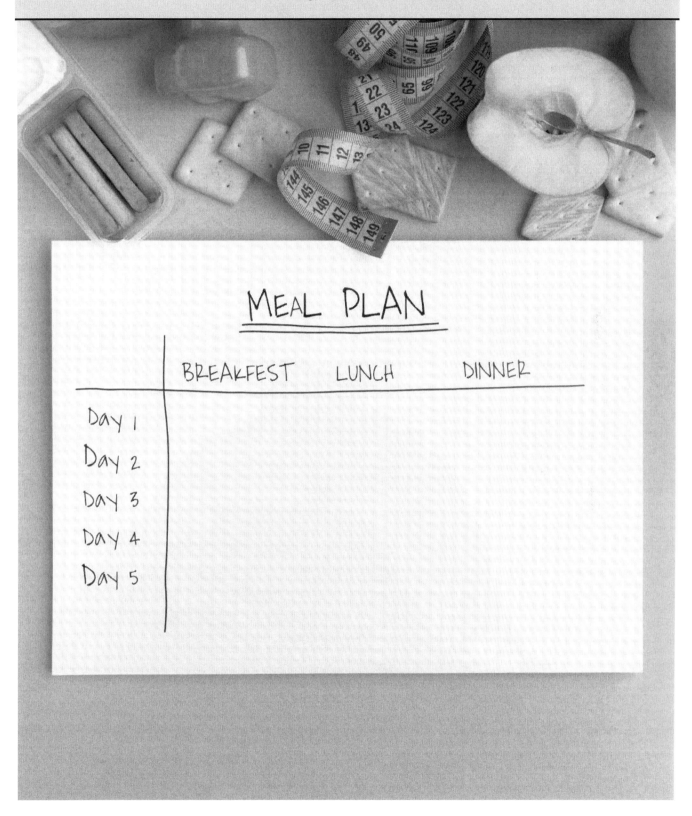

MEAL PLAN

	BREAKFEST	LUNCH	DINNER
Day 1			
Day 2			
Day 3			
Day 4			
Day 5			

Days	Breakfast	Lunch	Dinner
1	Berry Smoothie Bowl	Honey-Mustard Fruit-Sauced Chicken	Creamy asparagus soup
2	Overnight Cherry-Almond Oatmeal	Beef stew with fennel and shallots	Baked chicken and wild rice with onion and tarragon
3	Chicken and Asparagus Crepes	Roasted Root Veggies and Spiced Lentils	Brown Rice Tuna Bake
4	Banana Oatmeal Pancakes	Grilled chicken salad with olives and oranges	Grilled Veggie Subs
5	Apple Cinnamon Chia Pudding	Jerk Chicken with Mango salsa	Peasant Soup
6	Yogurt & Honey Fruit Cups	Lemony Chicken	Pasta primavera
7	Blueberry Muffins	Grilled chicken salad with olives and oranges	Squash and Rice Bake
8	Apple Pancakes	Buffalo Chicken Wrap	Tofu and Broccoli Stir-Fry
9	French Toast	Chicken tamales	Grilled Veggie Subs
10	Pumpkin Pie Oatmeal	Cream of Celery Soup	Juicy Burgers
11	Breakfast Parfaits	Grilled chicken salad with olives and oranges	Chicken and Dumplings
12	Overnight Peach Oatmeal	Brunswick Stew	Provençal Baked Fish with Roasted Potatoes & Mushrooms
13	Brunch-Style Portobello Mushrooms	French green lentil salad	Mango Shrimp Kebabs
14	Healthy Blueberry Smoothie with Almond Butter	Paella with chicken, leeks, and tarragon	Bean and Tomato Curry
15	Garlic-Herb Mini Quiches	Buffalo Chicken Wrap	Mexican Bean Bake
16	Oatmeal Waffles	Baked Tilapia in Garlic and Olive Oil	Vegetarian Bolognese
17	Banana Oat Breakfast Cookies	Grilled Southwestern Chicken Breasts	Carrot Rice

18	Breakfast Parfaits	Grilled chicken salad with olives and oranges	Chicken and Dumplings
19	Autumn Power Porridge	Chili Chicken Breasts	Brunswick Stew
20	Hummus and Date Bagel	White chicken chili	Mango Shrimp Kebabs
21	Pear-Stuffed French Vanilla Toast	Bean and Tomato Curry	Lebanese Chicken and Potatoes
22	Oatmeal Waffles	Baked Tilapia in Garlic and Olive Oil	Vegetarian Bolognese
23	Apple Pancakes	Buffalo Chicken Wrap	Tofu and Broccoli Stir-Fry
24	Berry Smoothie Bowl	Honey-Mustard Fruit-Sauced Chicken	Creamy asparagus soup
25	Breakfast Parfaits	Grilled chicken salad with olives and oranges	Chicken and Dumplings
26	Brunch-Style Portobello Mushrooms	French green lentil salad	Mango Shrimp Kebabs
27	Overnight Peach Oatmeal	Brunswick Stew	Provençal Baked Fish with Roasted Potatoes & Mushrooms
28	Pear-Stuffed French Vanilla Toast	Bean and Tomato Curry	Lebanese Chicken and Potatoes
29	Blueberry Muffins	Grilled chicken salad with olives and oranges	Squash and Rice Bake
30	Yogurt & Honey Fruit Cups	Lemony Chicken	

Mediterranean Diet
Cookbook
for
Beginners

1800 days of easy and delicious recipes for eating healthy and living well

GET YOUR BONUS NOW!

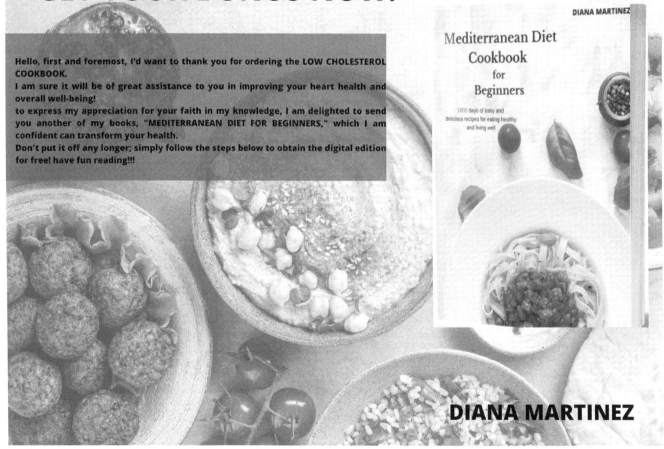

DIANA MARTINEZ

Mediterranean Diet Cookbook for Beginners

1800 days of easy and delicious recipes for eating healthy and living well

DIANA MARTINEZ

Conclusion

You're twice as likely to get heart disease if you have high cholesterol. This is why it's critical to get your cholesterol levels examined and regulated, particularly if you have a family history of heart disease.

This collection of recipes can help you establish a healthy lifestyle. After going through these recipes, you'll see that changing to a healthier lifestyle isn't that tough. You may have a diverse diet with nutrients and many recipes to select from. But the greatest part is that you'll get to taste all of the exquisite tastes and ingredients. This cookbook will undoubtedly transform your life, with everything from quick and simple stir fry meals to hearty breakfast ideas. There are also some dessert options when you want something healthy, sweet, and indulgent throughout the month.

It's a shift that can help everyone, from those who need to decrease their cholesterol to those who. Simply put, adopting a cholesterol-lowering diet and exercise routine lowers the risk of heart disease. Making this change is liberating. Finding new, healthier cooking methods that aren't expensive and don't taste or feel like a "diet" can be a lot of fun.

The purpose of this book is not to harp on and about the risks of cholesterol. Rather, it's about setting a plan that includes attainable objectives and simple, delicious foods. It's a step-by-step approach to get you started on a low-cholesterol lifestyle.

Made in the USA
Monee, IL
09 March 2023

29505976R10098